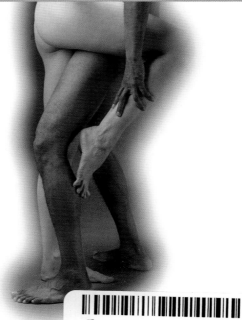

POSITION
SEX BIBLE

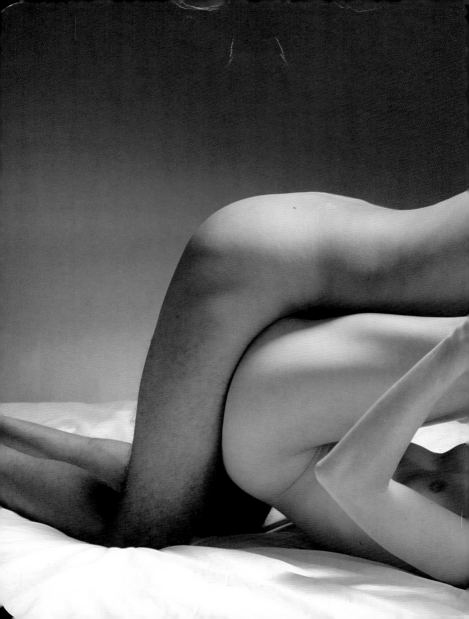

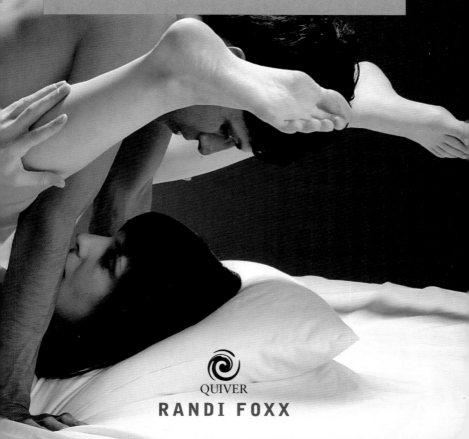

POSITION SEX BIBLE

MORE POSITIONS THAN YOU COULD POSSIBLY IMAGINE TRYING

QUIVER

RANDI FOXX

This 2008 edition published by
Quiver, a member of
Quarto Publishing Group USA Inc.
100 Cummings Center
Suite 406-L
Beverly, MA 01915-6101
www.quiverbooks.com

First published in 2004 by Hylas Publishing
129 Main Street, Suite C
Irvington, New York 10533
www.hylaspublishing.com

ISBN-13: 978-1-59233-349-3
ISBN-10: 1-59233-349-4

18 17 16 15 14   24 25 26 27

Cover Design: Carol Holtz
Publisher: Sean Moore
Publishing Director: Karen Price
Art Directors: Gus Yoo, Edwin Kuo
Editor: Angda Goel
Production Manager: Sarah Reilly
Photographer: Robert Wright

Printed and bound in Hong Kong

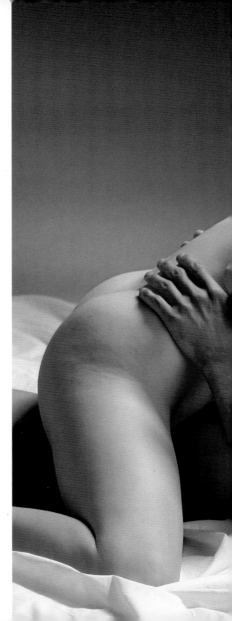

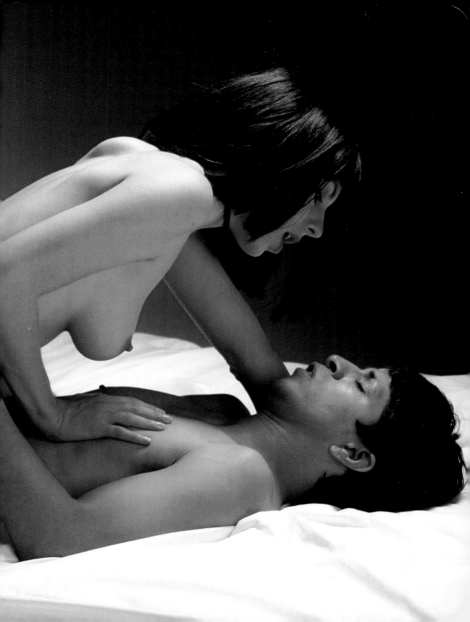

Contents

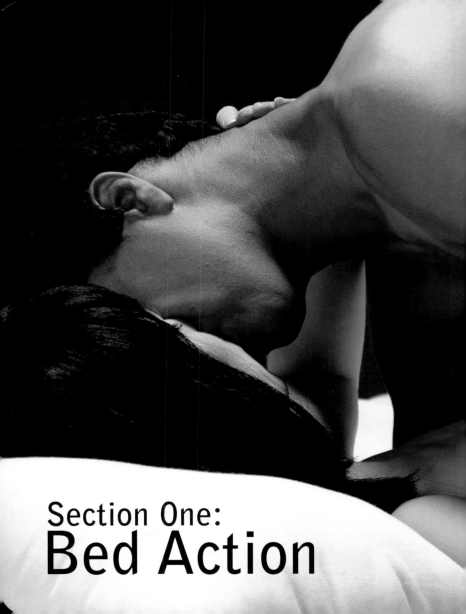

Section One:
Bed Action

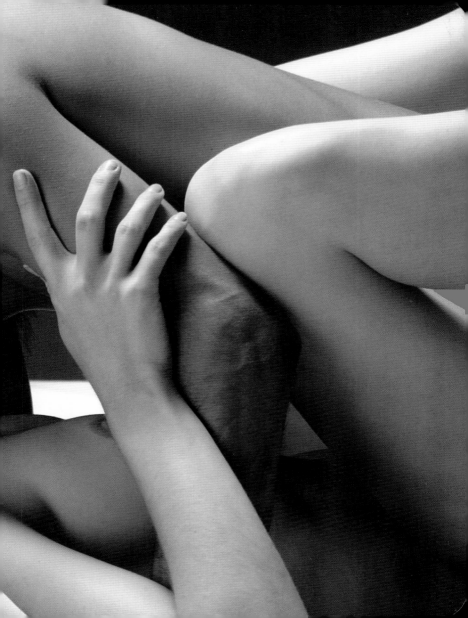

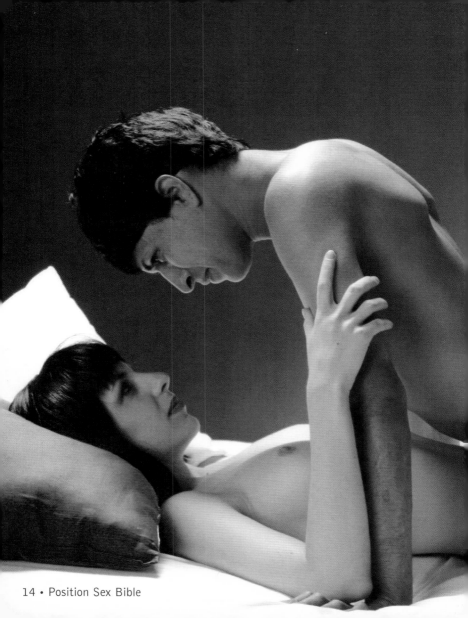

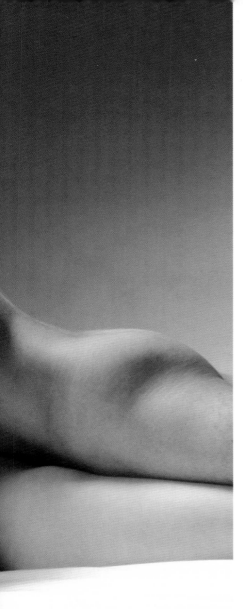

Straight-Edge Sex A

Most commonly known as the Missionary Position; also called the Clasping position. The man is on top and the legs of both the man and woman are stretched out straight. The partners face one another.

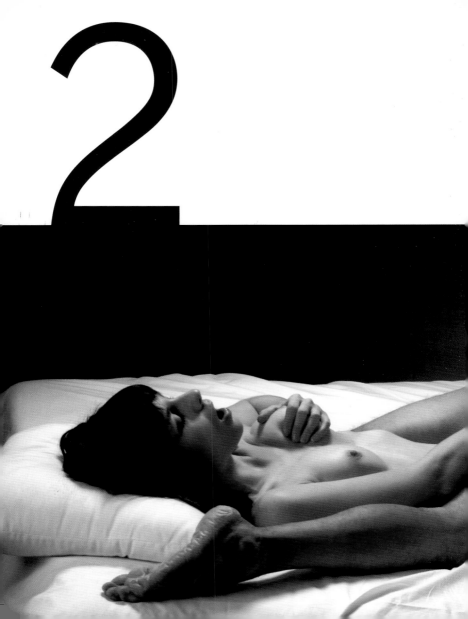

Foot Rub with Rhythm

In Straight-Edge Sex A (1), the man turns a full 360° while in union. When he is 180° to his partner, he can stop to give her a nice foot massage! (She can take this opportunity to caress his buttocks and get a new view of her lover's body). It takes a lot of practice to do this move without the penis slipping out repeatedly, but the angles of penetration are worth it!

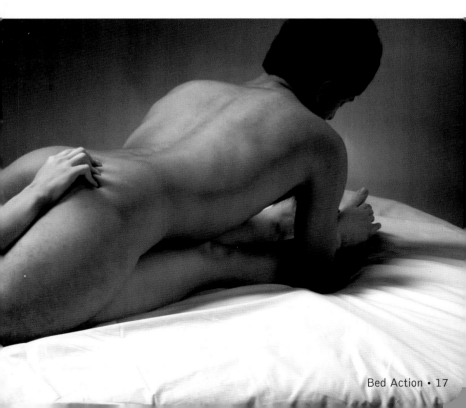

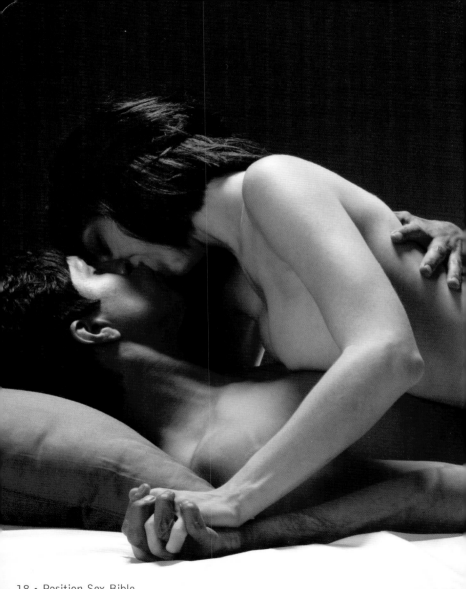

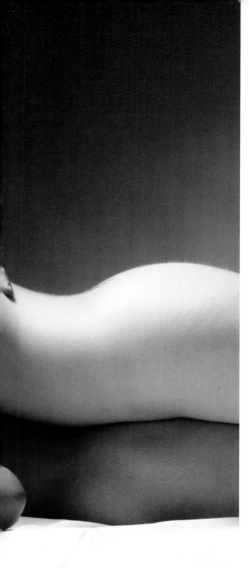

3

Straight-Edge Sex B

Straight-Edge Sex A (1),
but with the woman on top.

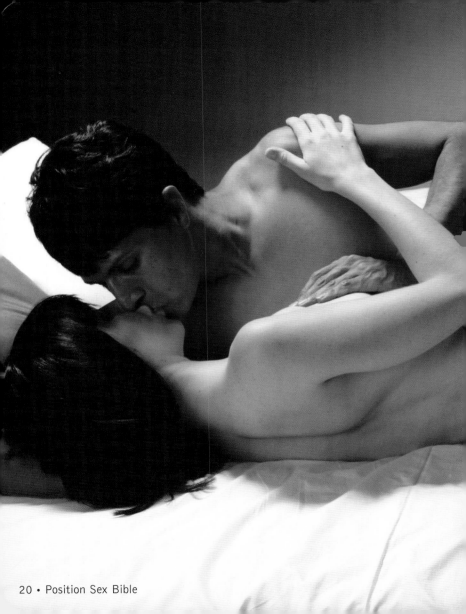

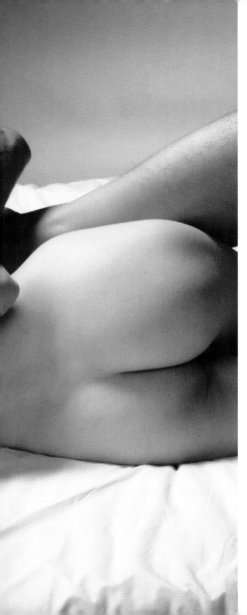

4

Always by Your Side

Variation of Straight-Edge Sex, with both partners face to face, but on their sides. A hand is then free to explore the rest of your lover's body.

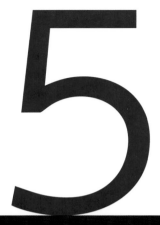

5

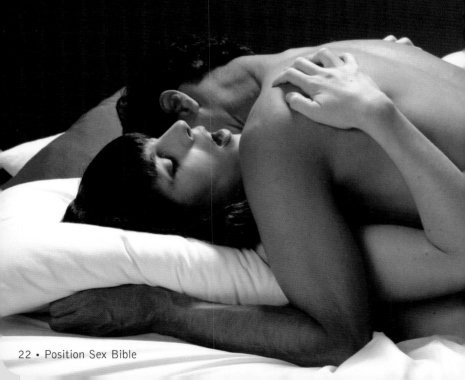

Pig in a Blanket

The most natural progression from Straight-Edge Sex A (1)
While the man is on top, the woman wraps her legs
around his waist, pulling him into her more.

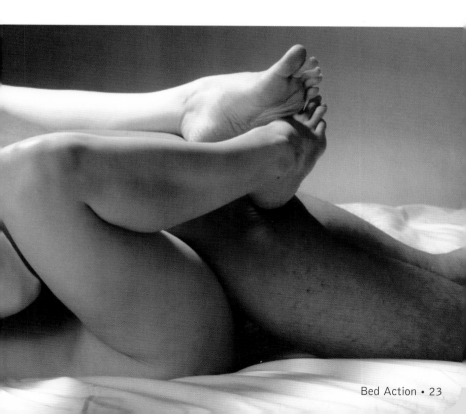

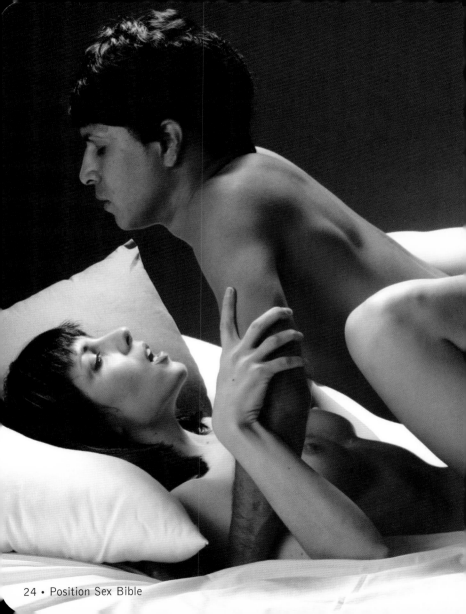

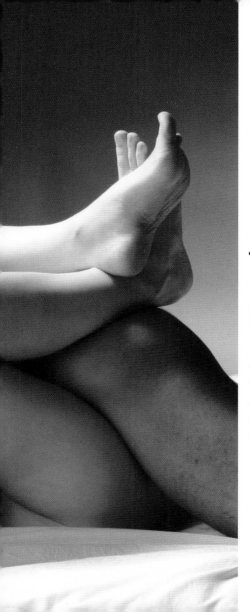

6

The Penitent Forgiven

A slight shift from the Pig in a Blanket (5); the legs of the woman are still wrapped around the man (who is on top), but the man is kneeling with his arms at her sides.

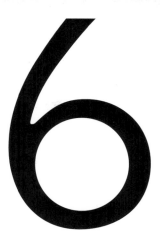

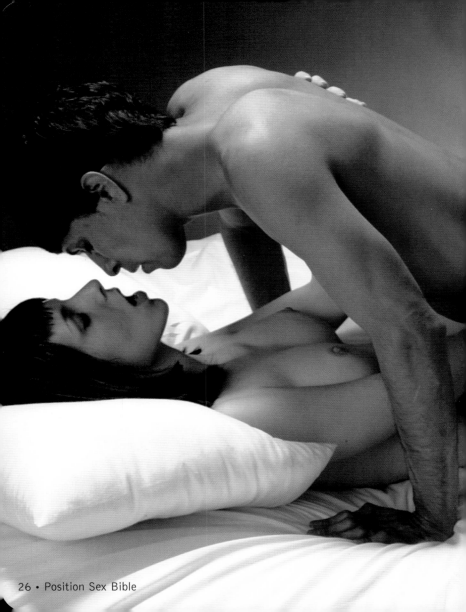

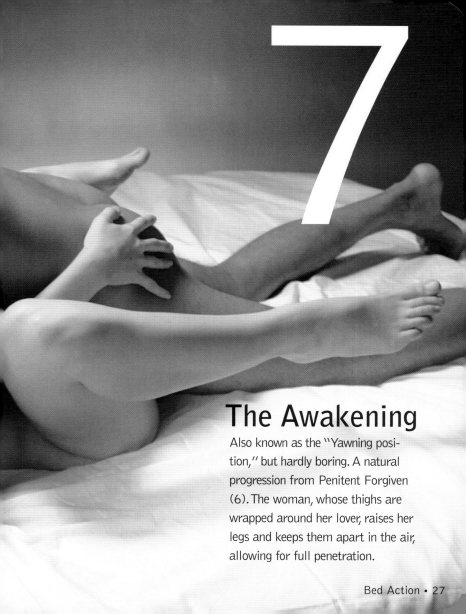

The Awakening

Also known as the "Yawning position," but hardly boring. A natural progression from Penitent Forgiven (6). The woman, whose thighs are wrapped around her lover, raises her legs and keeps them apart in the air, allowing for full penetration.

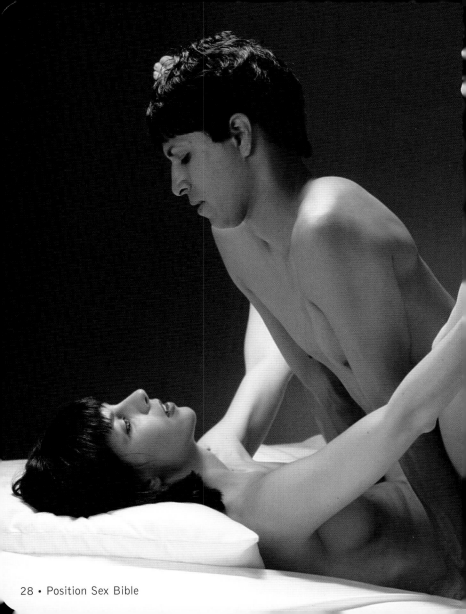

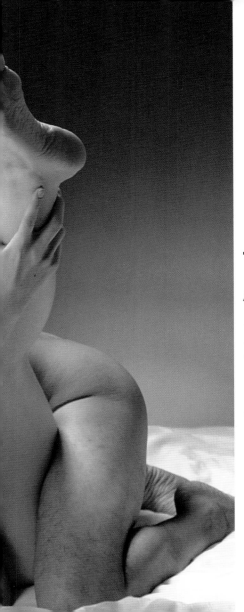

8

The Piked Awakening

Acrobatic variation of the Awakening (7); the woman throws her raised legs back in a pike position and lifts her vagina, allowing for full and deep penetration. For better control, she can hold her calves with her hands. (A pillow under her lower back also helps). The man, who is on top, relies mostly on upper-body strength and can lie or kneel over the woman.

9
Inner Awakening

Variation of Awakening (7), with the legs of the woman on the inside of the man's arms, allowing her to rest her legs on his shoulders, or to bend them back over his arms. This position is more comfortable for the woman than the Awakening, and can be sustained for longer. She also has better access to his buttocks and face.

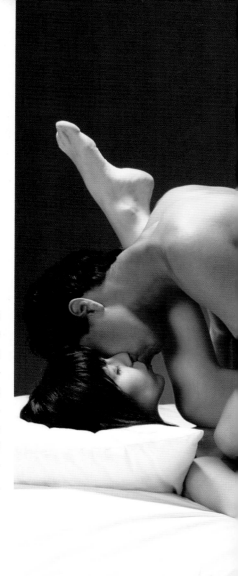

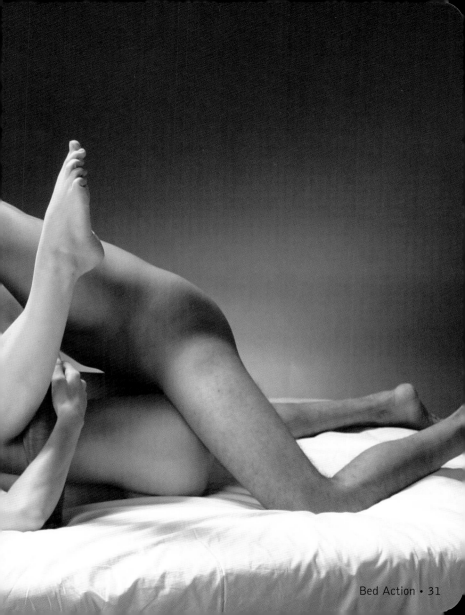

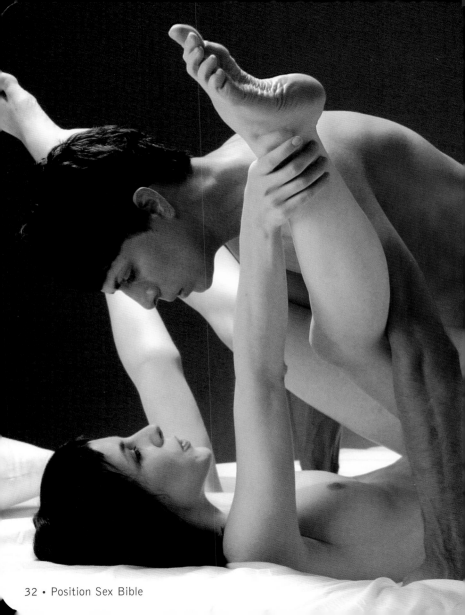

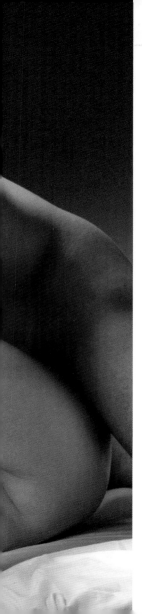

10

Scissors

Similar to Splitting of a Bamboo (11); while on her back, the woman moves her legs back and forth in the air while penetrated by her kneeling lover. This motion squeezes the penis, causing powerful sensations for both partners.

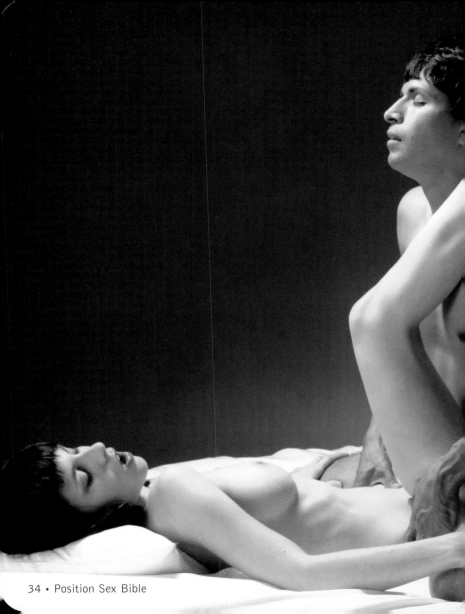

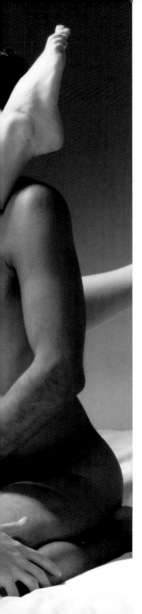

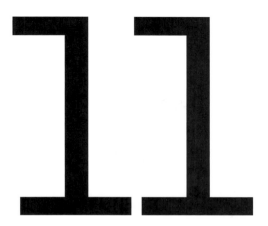

11

Splitting of a Bamboo

Straight from the **Kama Sutra**—an easy progression from the Inner Awakening (9). The woman uses the motion of her legs to squeeze the penis while it is in the vagina. A single leg rises onto her partner's shoulder and then lowers; the other leg repeats this motion.

12

Hammerhead

Variation of Splitting of a Bamboo (11); the act is similar to hammering in a nail— while the man kneels and thrusts forward, the woman places her foot on his forehead instead of on his shoulder.

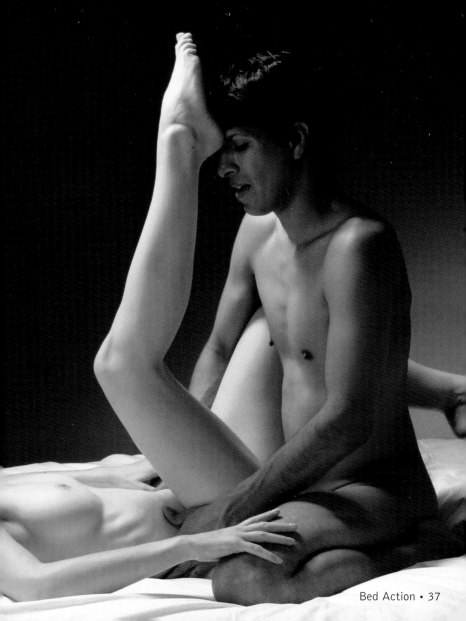

Bed Action • 37

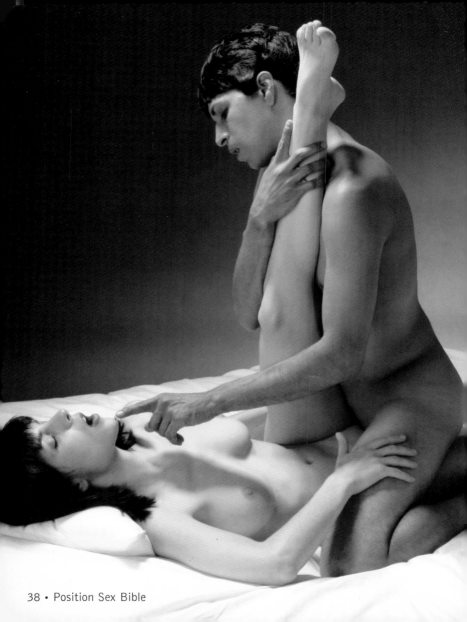

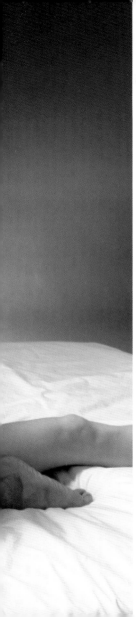

13

Jackknifed Splits

Similar to Splitting of a Bamboo (11), but the woman has one leg under her kneeling lover and the other raised across his body, resting against his face. From this vantage point, the man can see his penis thrust in and out of the vagina, and the woman's breasts undulate in rhythm to the motion.

14

Lateral Jackknifed Splits

In a natural move from Jackknifed Splits (13), the woman's leg comes over the side of her partner, resting against his thigh. This position is the perfect prelude to the Elephant (74).

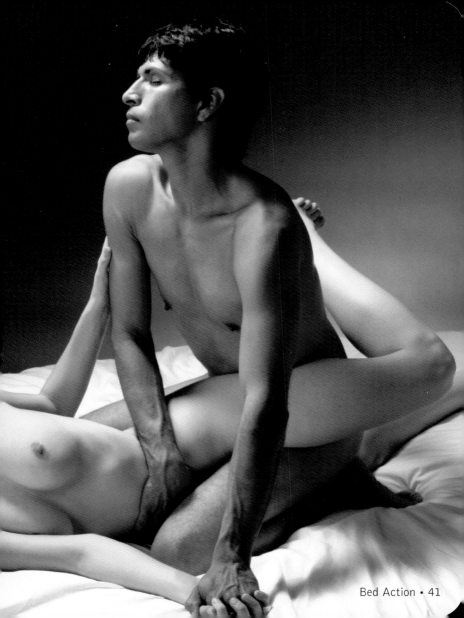

15

Climbing Ivy

The man kneels while facing his lover who lies on her back. She raises her legs and wraps them around his neck, allowing for deep penetration. He can take hold of her thighs and guide himself into her.

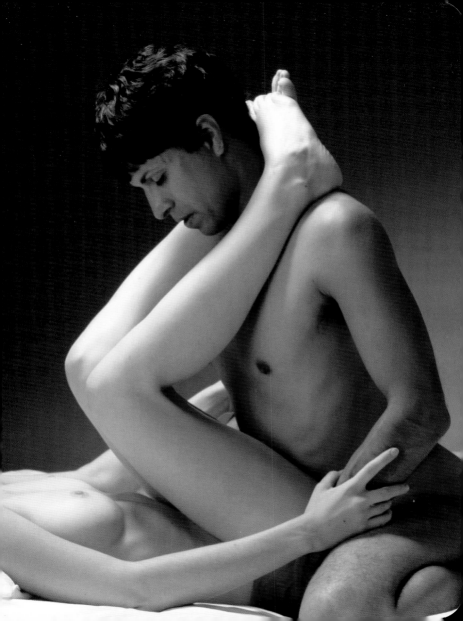

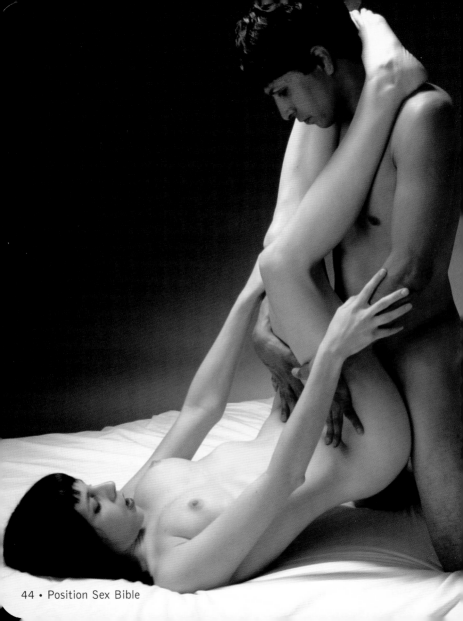

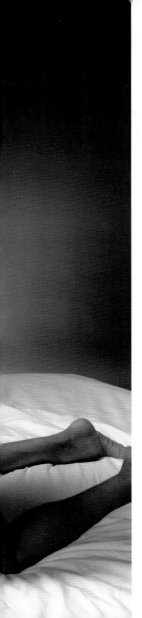

16

Inverted Wheelbarrow

An extreme variation of Climbing Ivy (15); the woman is almost upside-down, with only her head and neck on the bed. Her legs are on either side of her lover's head, and her lower back and buttocks are in the air. She may want to hold onto his thighs for support, and he will have to hold her legs while inside of her.

17

The Crab

Moving from the Awakening (7), the man takes a more dominating role and the woman pulls herself into a ball, with her legs folded against her chest. The man straddles her while kneeling, allowing for deep penetration.

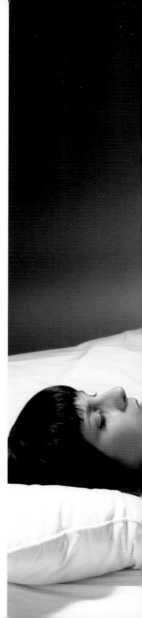

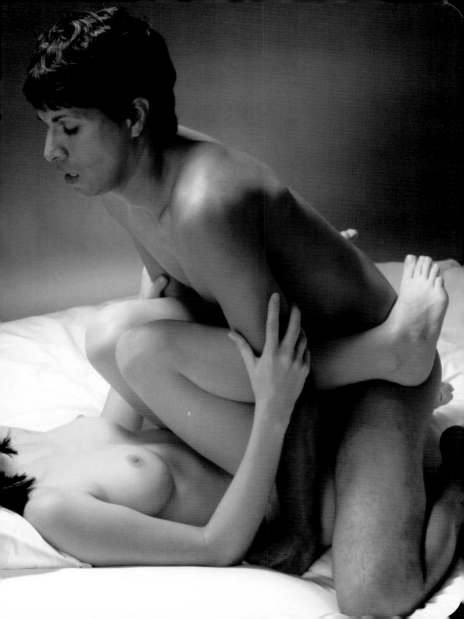

18

The Wrapped Crab

The man crouches on the balls of his feet, and the woman, on her back, moves from the Crab (17) and wraps her legs over his thighs.

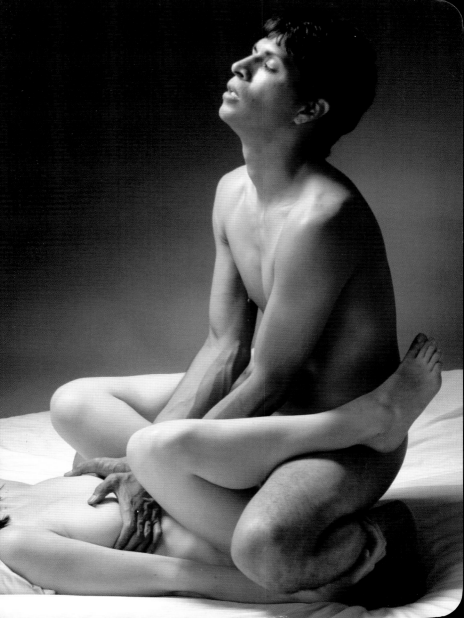

19

The Open Crab

Instead of pushing the folded legs against her chest, the woman opens her legs and rests her feet on her lover's thighs. Her vagina is fully open and her breasts are also exposed. The man is in control and can add to his dominance by pushing down on her shoulders.

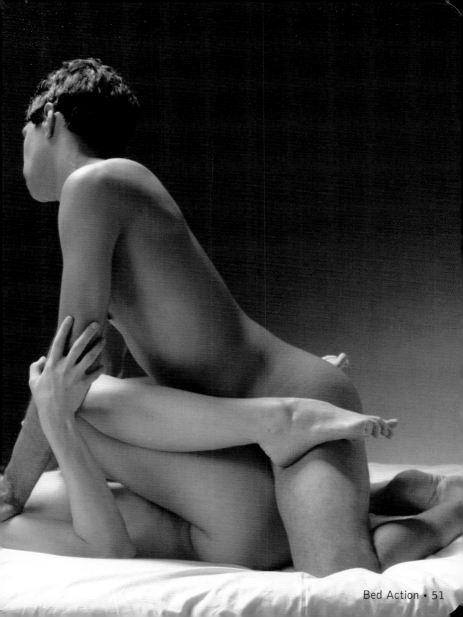

20

The Press

The woman is on her back and presses her feet against her partner's chest. He faces her while sitting up on his back legs, allowing for deep penetration.

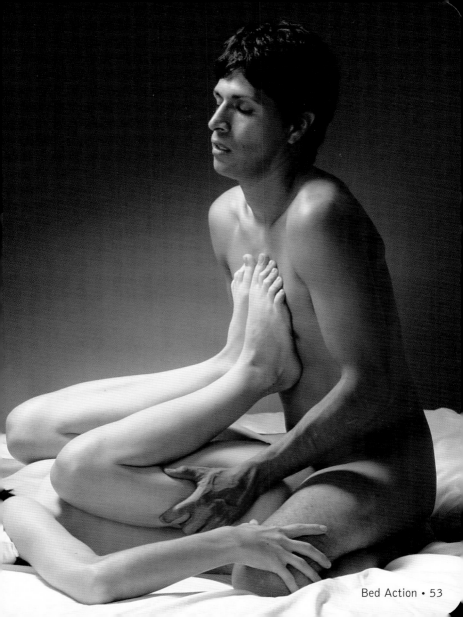

21

The Bicycle

Similar to Splitting of a Bamboo (11); the woman presses one foot against her lover's chest and raises the other leg in the air, as though she were riding a bicycle.

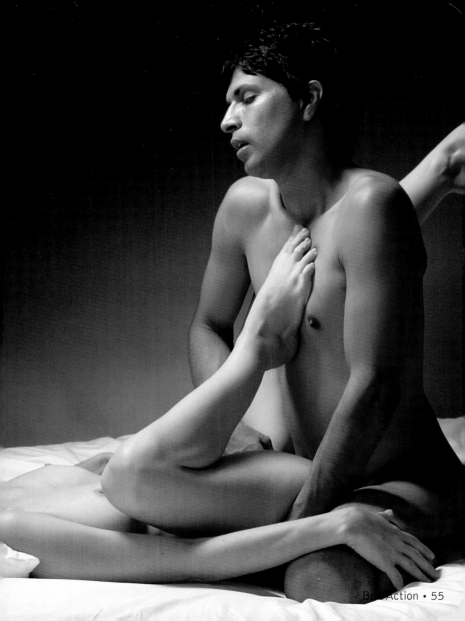

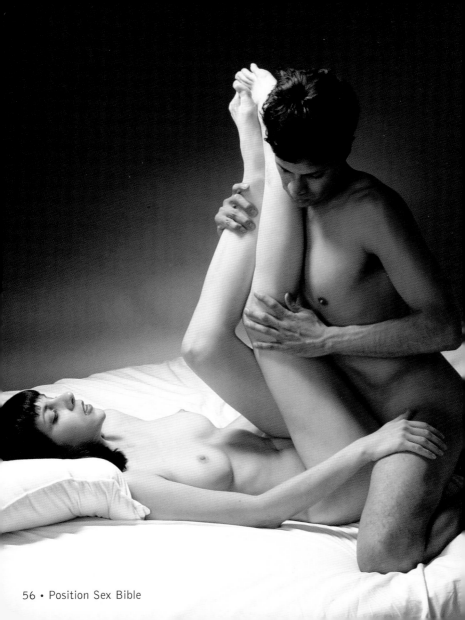

22

Side-to-Side Press

Variation of the Press (20); the man takes his lover's ankles, removes them from his chest, and shifts them from one side of his body to the other. This motion causes her vaginal muscles to contract around the penis. At the same time, he can kiss and caress her legs, ankles, and feet.

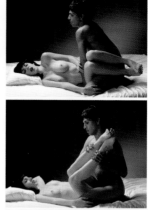
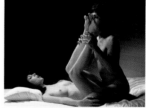
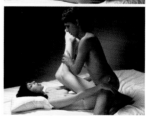
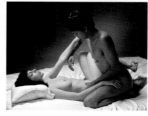

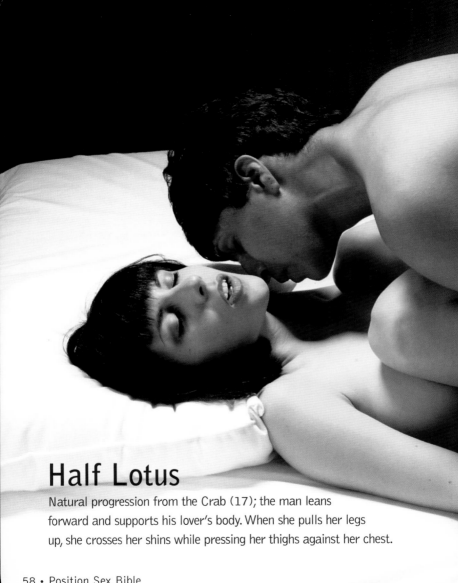

Half Lotus

Natural progression from the Crab (17); the man leans forward and supports his lover's body. When she pulls her legs up, she crosses her shins while pressing her thighs against her chest.

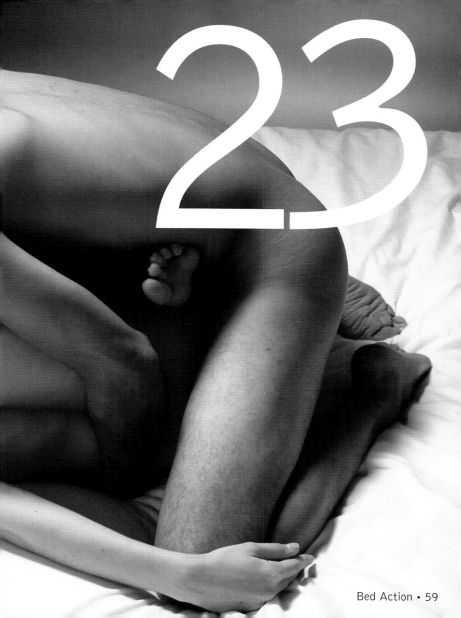

23

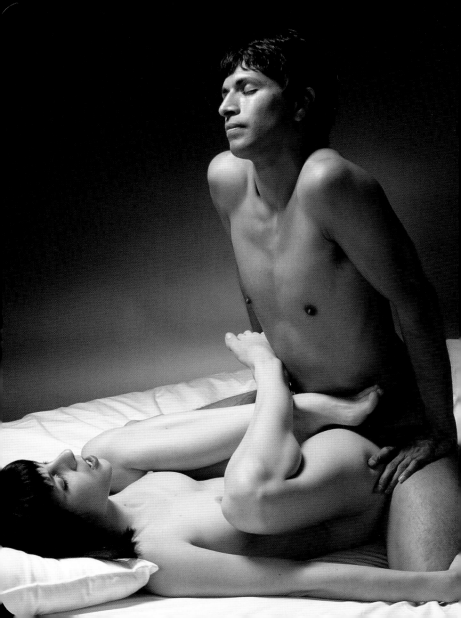

24

Full Lotus

Takes the lotus position of yoga and brings it into the bedroom. The woman assumes this position while on her back with her legs folded above her. Her partner leans forward and enters her while facing her and resting back on his legs.

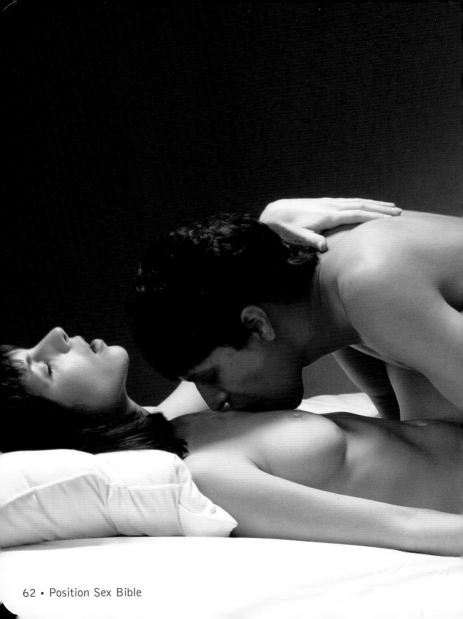

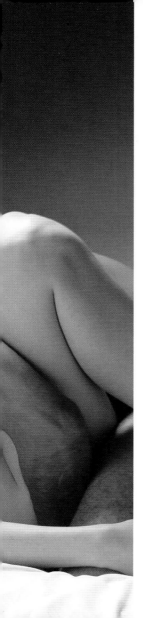

25

Wife of Indra

Extreme variation of the Crab (17); the woman pushes her legs back and to her sides instead of letting them rest against her chest. This position fully opens the vagina to the man for deep penetration.

26

Kneel and Extend

The woman lies on her back and pulls in her knees. The man kneels in front of her and enters her. She then extends both legs to one of his shoulders. This position allows him to caress her thighs.

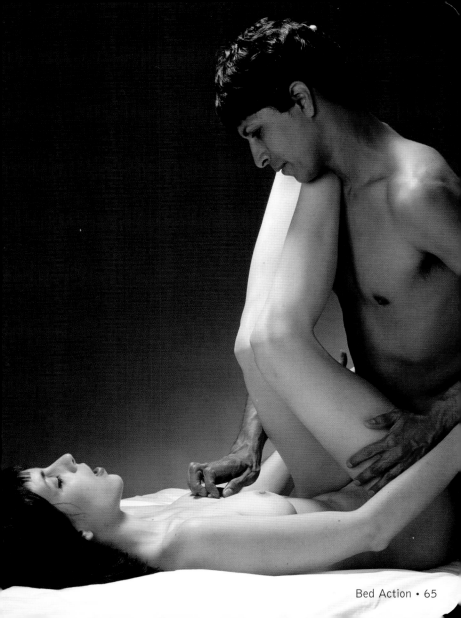

27

Lateral Kneel and Extend

Instead of raising her legs to her lover's shoulder, while on her back, the woman drapes her legs over one of his thighs. The man sits back on his legs and faces her. From this vantage point, he can see her getting aroused and may stroke her clitoris and breasts.

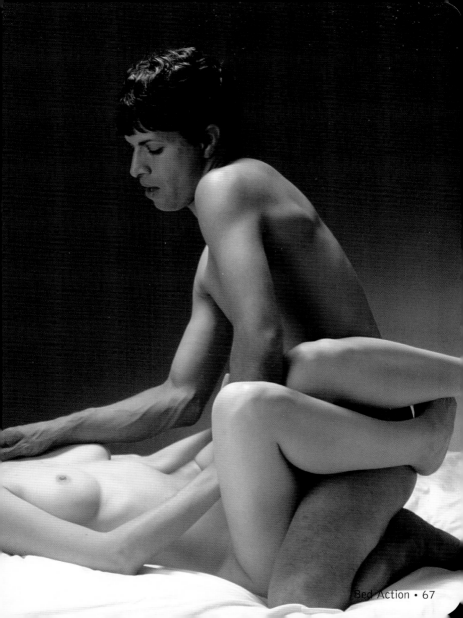

28

Kneel and Push Back

Variation of the Kneel and Extend (26);
instead of letting her legs rest on his shoulder,
the man holds them away from him, altering
the angle of penetration.

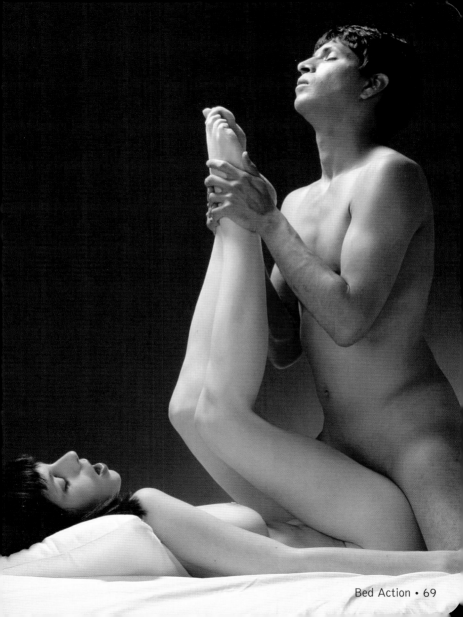

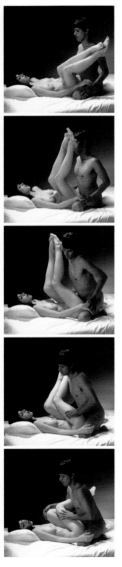

Side-to-Side Kneel and Extend

Variation of the Lateral Kneel and Extend (27); the woman swivels her legs back and forth from one of her lover's thighs to the other. This angle works well for G-spot arousal.

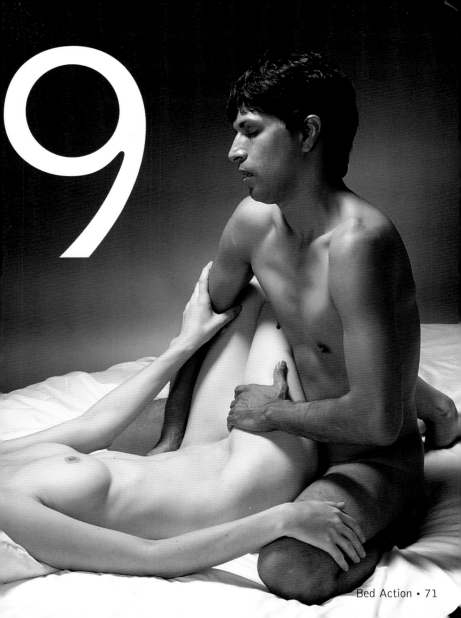

9

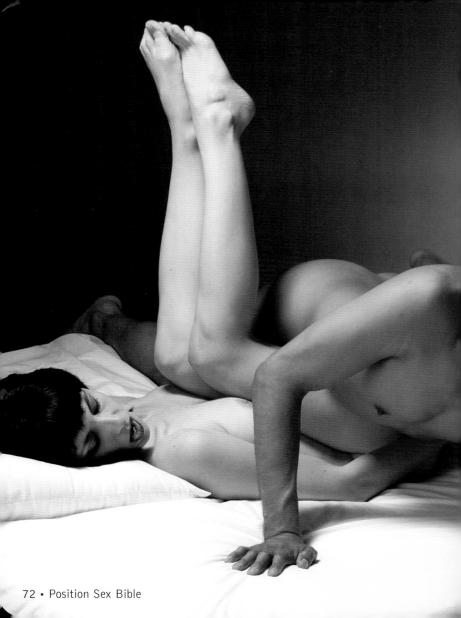

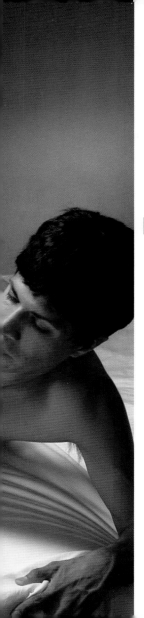

30

Surf's Up

The woman lies on her back with her legs extended above her. The man lies across her, preparing to catch the next wave of pleasure.

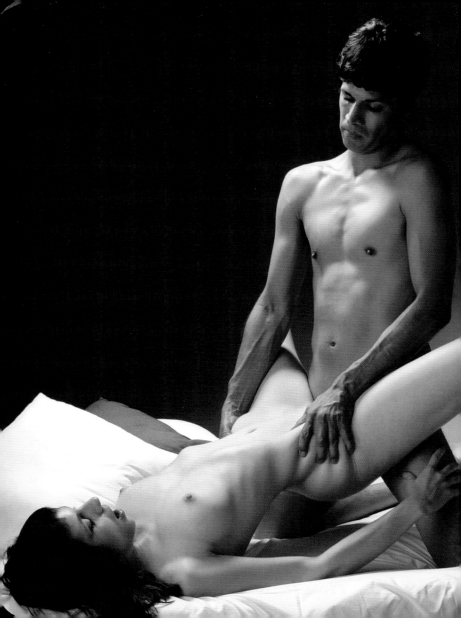

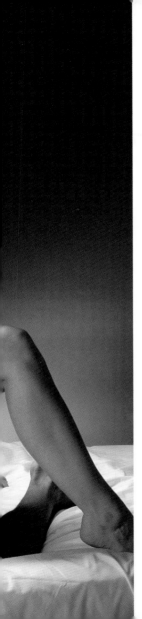

31

The Pelvic Thrust

From Straight-Edge Sex A (1), the woman moves her legs apart so that they are on the outside of the man's legs. The woman lowers her head, and raises her pelvis toward her partner. In this position, the vagina is fully open, allowing for deep penetration.

Pelvic Lap Dance

While on her back, the woman places her feet down and thrusts her pelvis up toward the man who is sitting on his hind legs. Similar to the Pelvic Thrust (31) with one important difference: the woman's buttocks are resting on her lover's thighs. While the woman arches her back, the man has full access to her stomach and breasts.

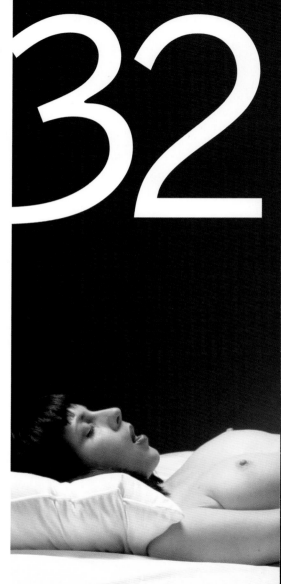

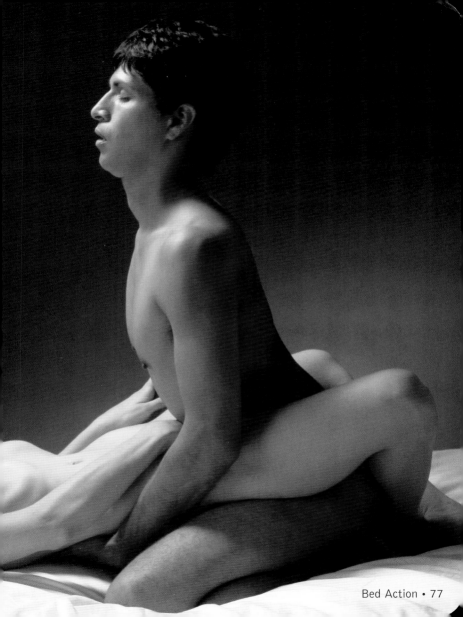

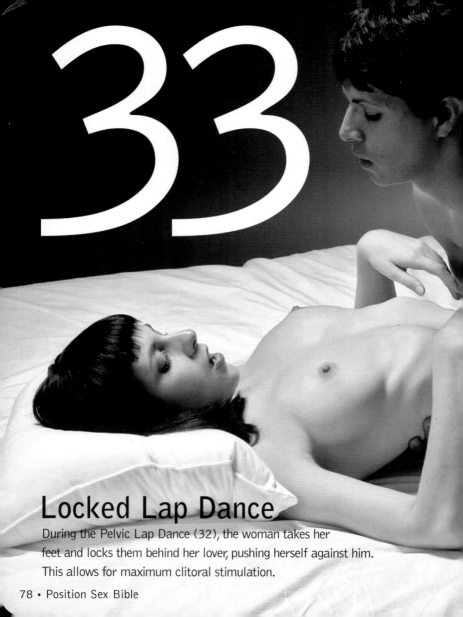

33

Locked Lap Dance

During the Pelvic Lap Dance (32), the woman takes her
feet and locks them behind her lover, pushing herself against him.
This allows for maximum clitoral stimulation.

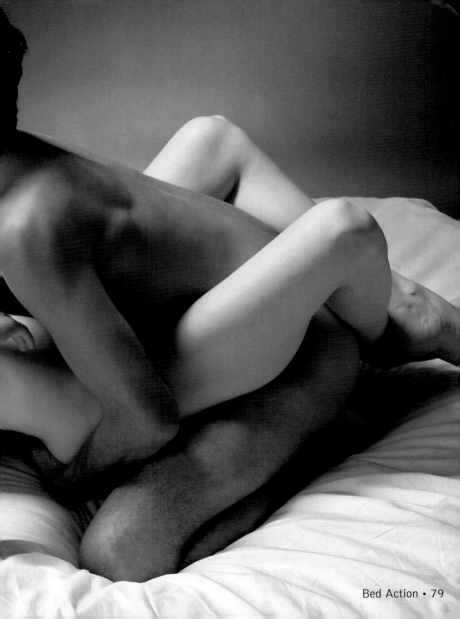

34

Kama's Wheel

Both partners sit facing one another, with the woman on the man's lap. The man sits with his legs outstretched and his lover mirrors his position (thus creating the spokes of a wheel with their legs).

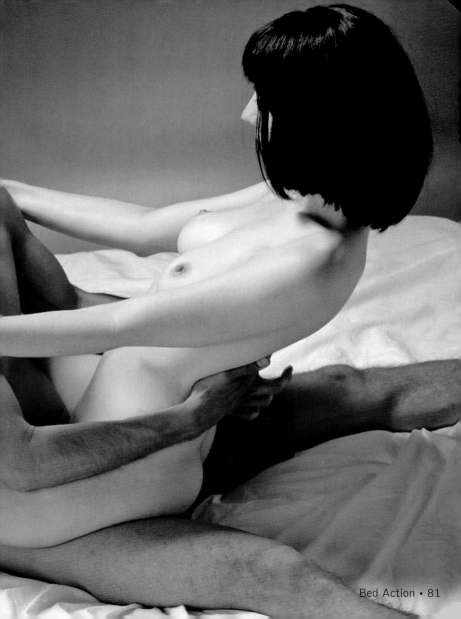

35

Reclining
Kama's Wheel

While in the Kama's Wheel (34), the woman leans
back on her elbows, altering the angle of penetration.
Her legs wrap around the back of her partner.

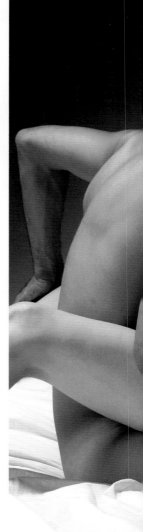

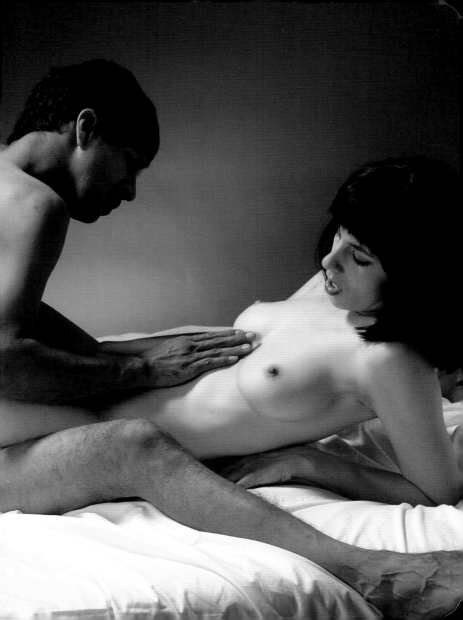

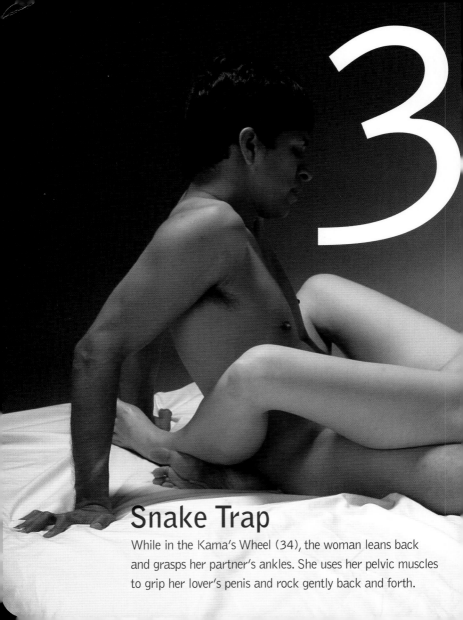

3

Snake Trap

While in the Kama's Wheel (34), the woman leans back
and grasps her partner's ankles. She uses her pelvic muscles
to grip her lover's penis and rock gently back and forth.

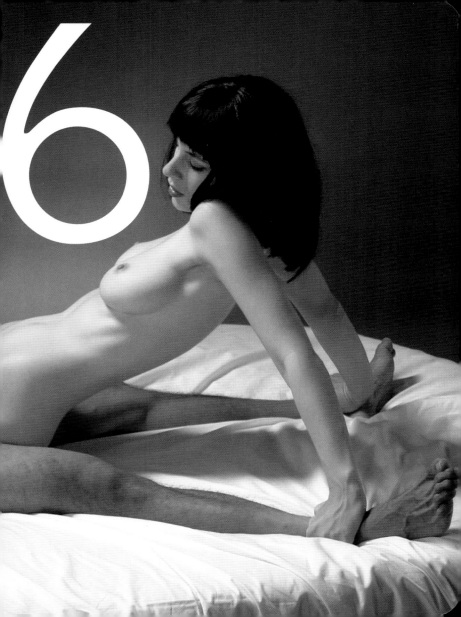

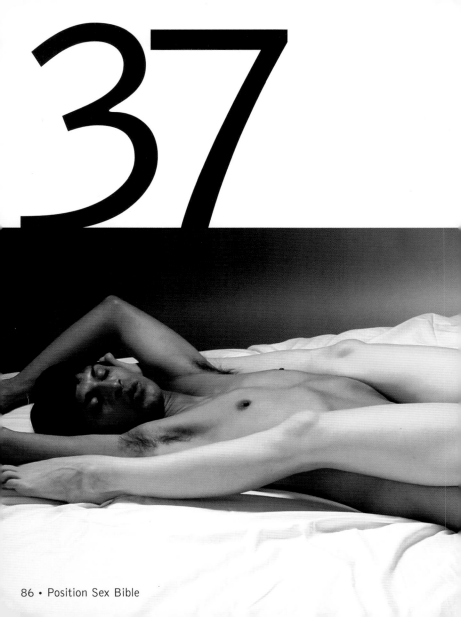

37

Full Reclining Snake Trap

Both lovers lean back while in the Kama's Wheel (34), forcing
the woman to use her vaginal muscles to maintain his erection.
The couple focuses on stimulating their subtle energy bodies
rather than their physical bodies—very tantric!

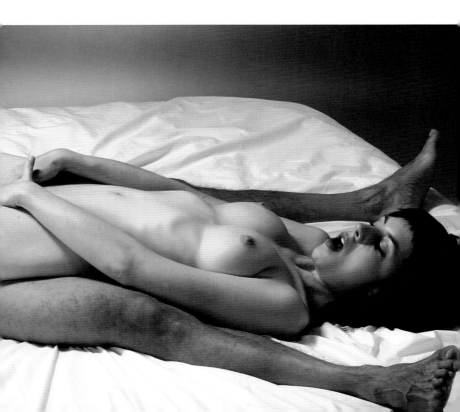

38

The Neverending Hug

The lovers sit face to face, straddling each
other's bodies. A position that allows for deep
penetration, kissing, and eye contact.

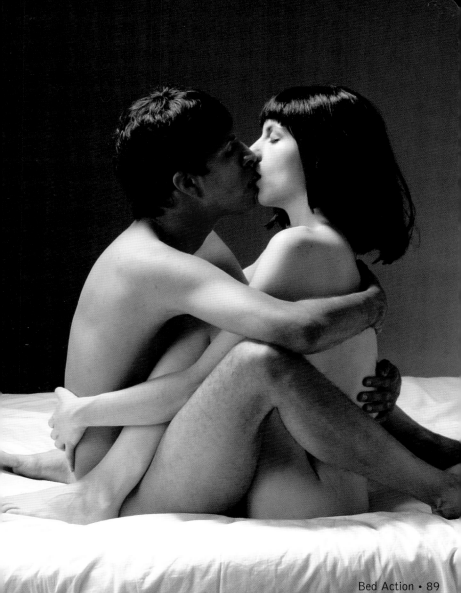

39

Paired Feet

From the Kama's Wheel (34), the woman leans
back and draws her legs up so that her shins are
resting on her partner's chest. The man opens his
legs wide apart, with her body between them, so
that the woman can experience full penetration.
Then he presses her thighs together to intensify
the sensations.

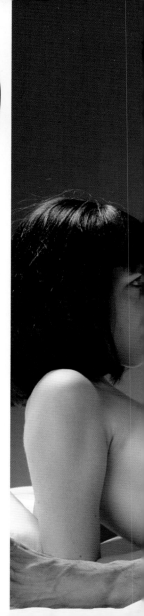

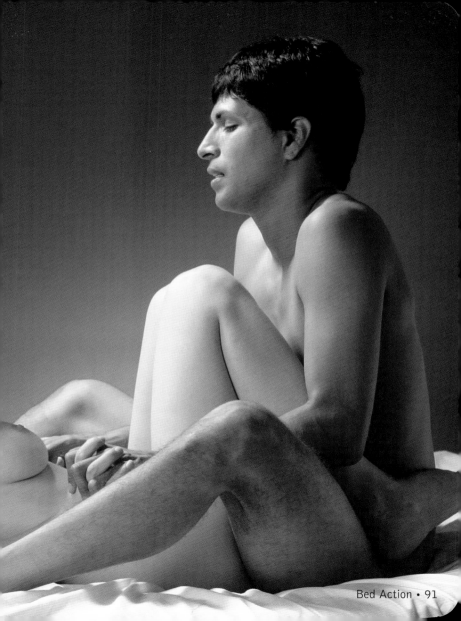

40

"X" Marks the Spot

Combination of the Full Reclining Snake Trap (37) and the Jackknifed Splits (13); the woman lies on her side with her legs apart. The man lies back with his legs apart. They meet in the middle, with one of her legs underneath him and her feet beside his face if he lies back.

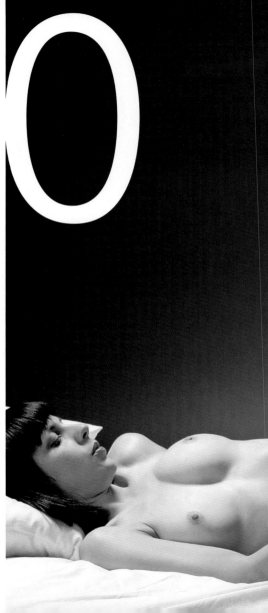

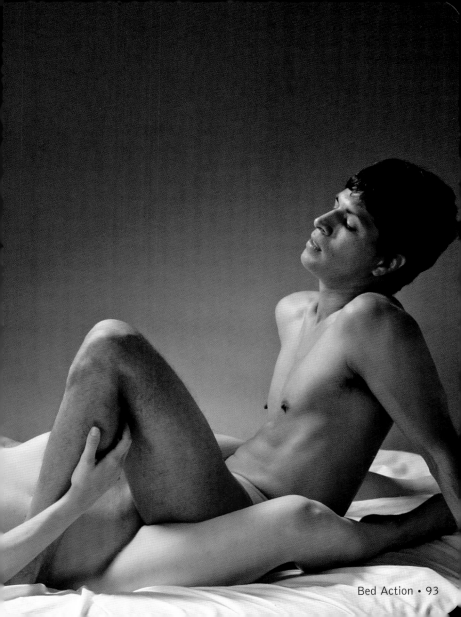

41

The Mare's Trick

More of a technique than a position, this method allows the woman to forcibly hold the man's penis in her vagina. She can usually achieve this by pressing her legs together. Best during Straight-Edge Sex B (3), where the woman is on top and can better control the action.

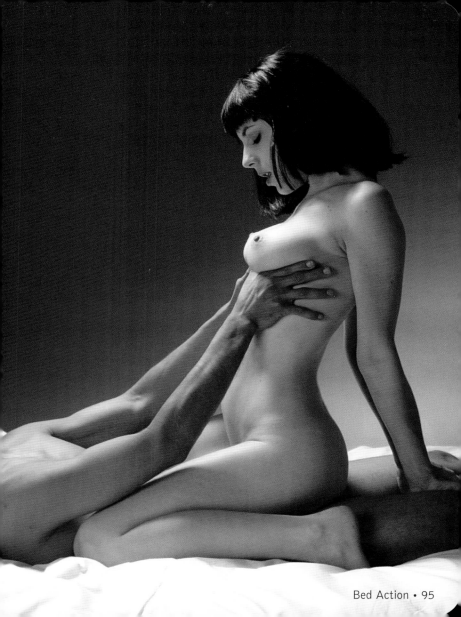

Pair of Tongs

Similar to the Mare's Trick (41); it is more of a sexual technique than a position. Once again, the woman straddles the man, who is facing her while lying on his back. The woman holds the penis in her vagina—drawing it in, pressing it and keeping it in for a long time. Intense eye contact and the woman stroking her lover's chest and testicles enhance this technique.

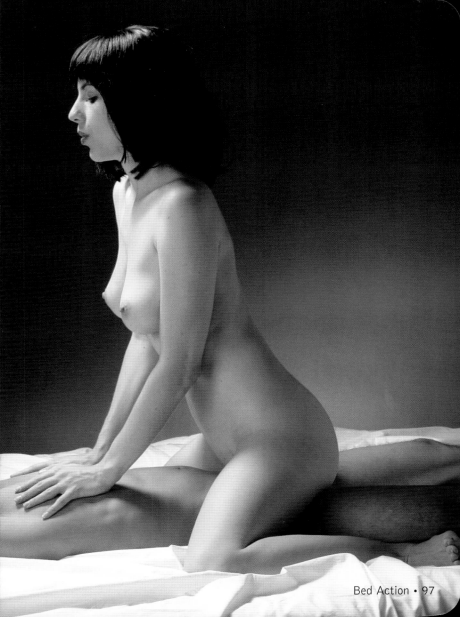

The Spinner

From the Bucking Bronco (51),
the woman rotates 360°,
experiencing every angle of
penetration. She has the
potential for G-spot activation
while her back is to her lover.
Perfect for smaller women
with larger partners.

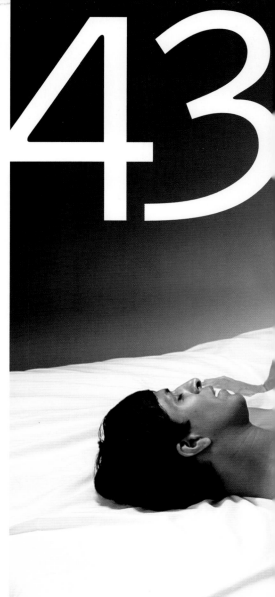

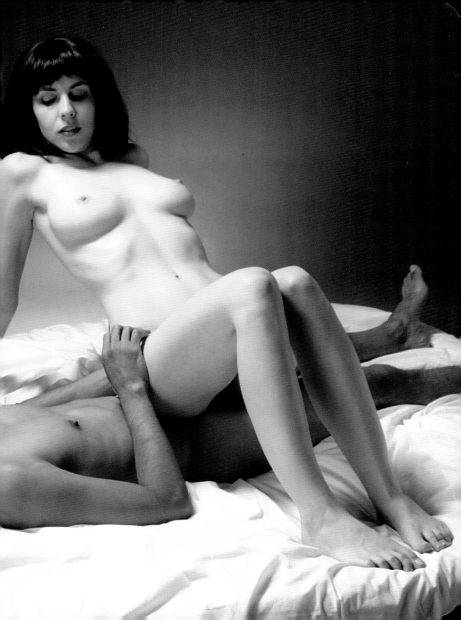

44

Back to Meditating

As the man lies on his back, his partner sits on him cross-legged with her back to him. Although there is little eye contact, the angle of entry is perfect for G-spot activation.

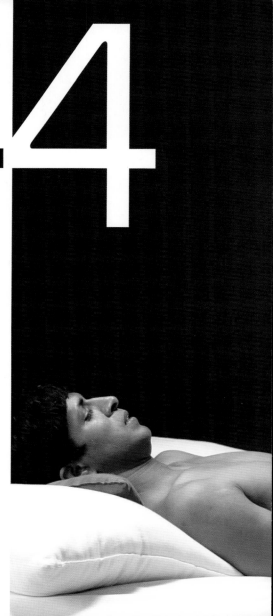

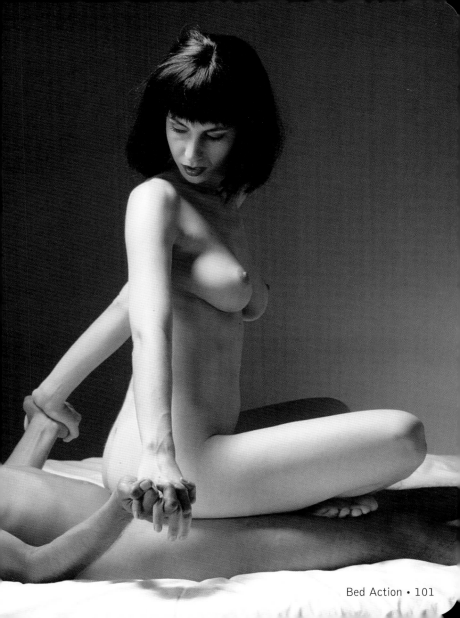

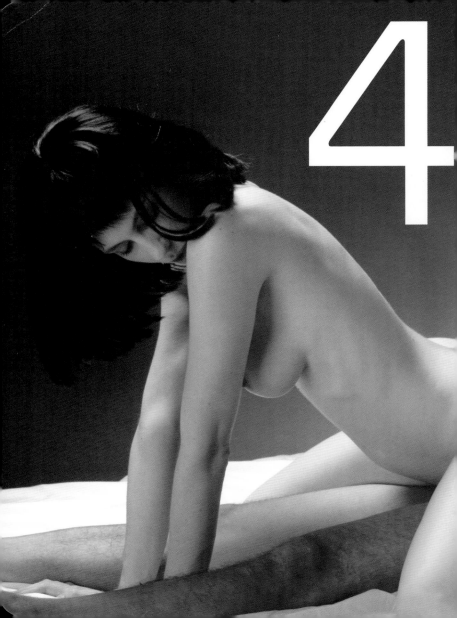

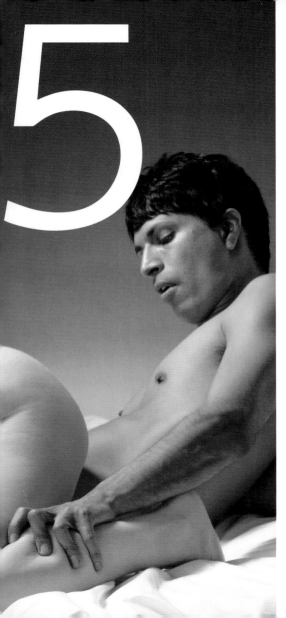

The Pin

The counterpart to Foot Rub with Rhythm (2); from Straight-Edge Sex B (3), the woman turns 180° and has her body between his legs while she rests on her hands (he is still on his back). Her legs straddle his.

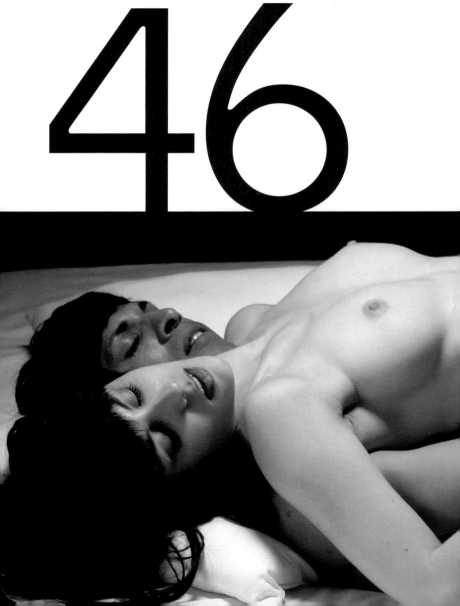

Spoon-on-Spoon

Variation on part of the Spinner sequence (43); while the woman has her back to the man, she lies on top of him. This allows him to run his hands all over her body, concentrating on her clitoris.

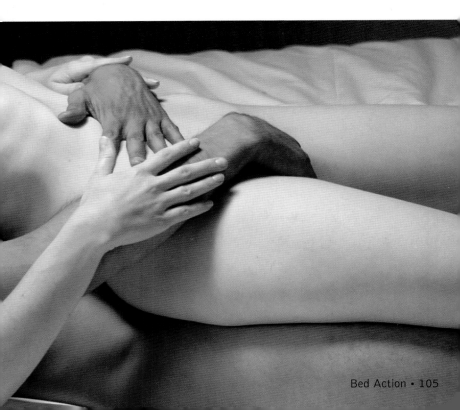

47

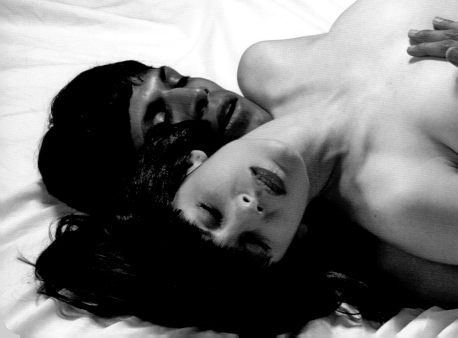

Stretched
Spoon-on-Spoon

From the Spoon-on-Spoon (46), the woman bends her
legs back, increasing the angle of penetration and the
opportunity for clitoral stimulation.

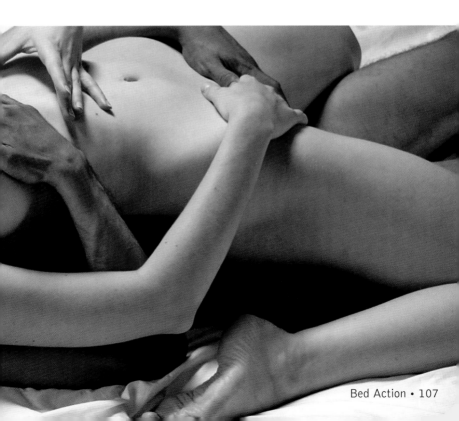

48

Sliding Into Home

Variation of the Bucking Bronco (51); the man's knees are bent so that the woman slides into him while on top of him. She can lean back onto his thighs as she rides him, leaving one hand free.

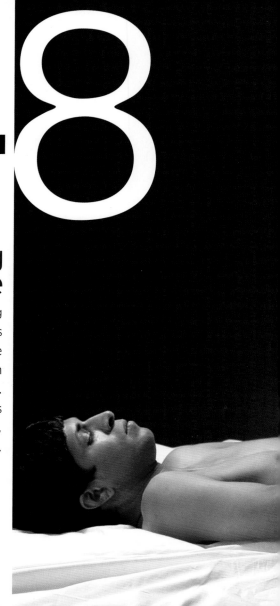

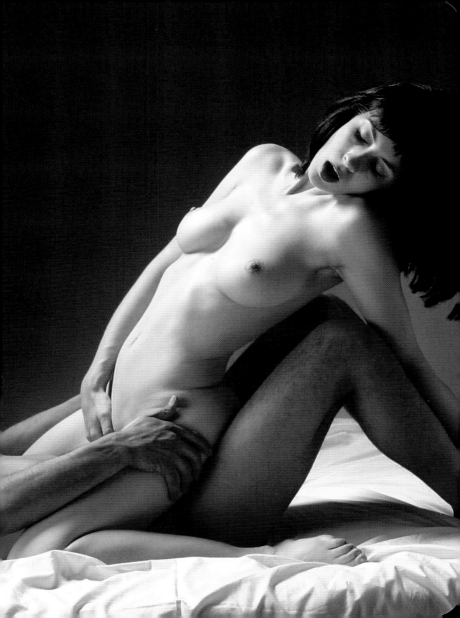

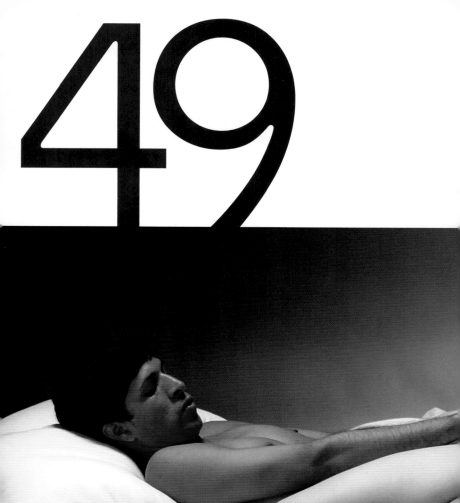

49

The Recliner

Another variation of the Bucking Bronco (51); while sitting and facing the man, the woman leans back onto her elbows. Her back is arched and he has full access to her clitoris. In this position, she can push his penis against the wall of her vagina.

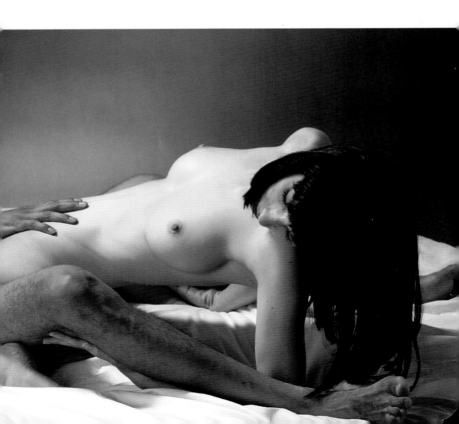

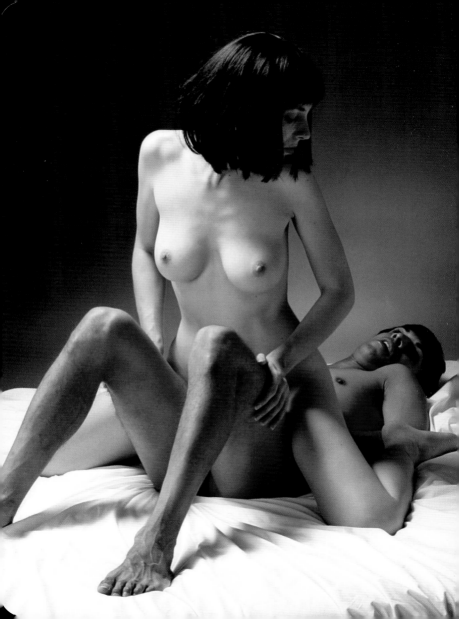

50

The Wrap Around

A shift from Sliding Into Home (48); the woman has her back to her lover and wraps her arms around his thighs as she sits straddles him.

51

The Bucking Bronco

The man lies on his back while the woman straddles her lover, facing him. She sits on him and rides him back and forth, and can place her hands on his chest while doing so. He has full access to her breasts and both partners can stimulate the clitoris.

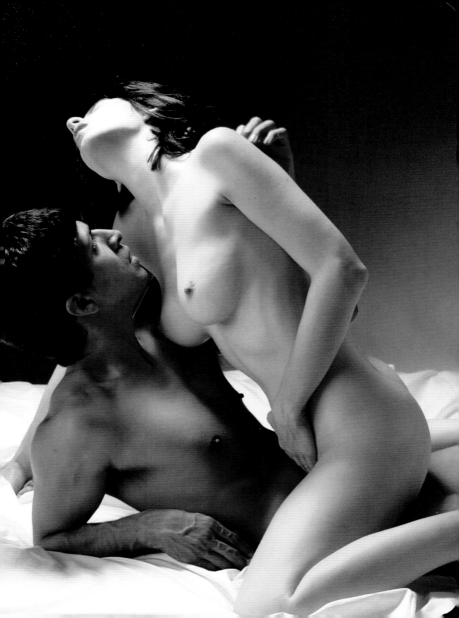

52

Will You Do Me?

The man kneels on one bended knee as though he were going to propose and enters his partner who faces him while kneeling with her legs apart.

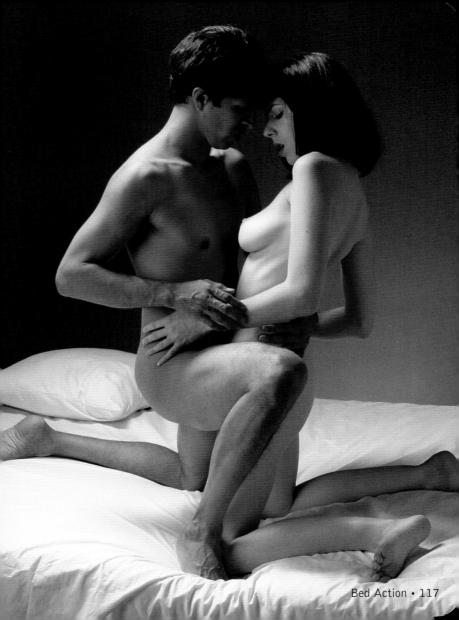

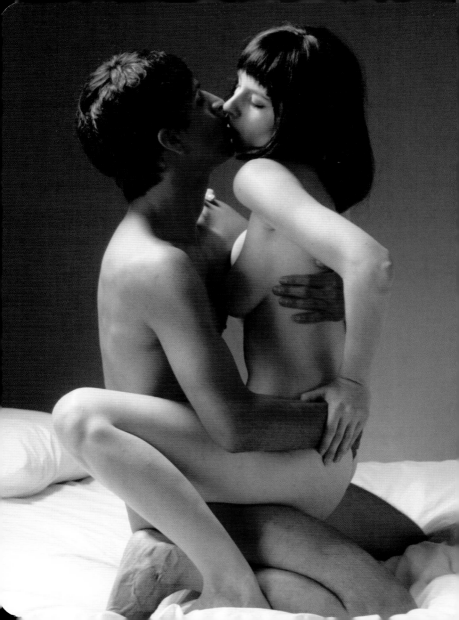

53

Crouching Tiger, Hidden Passion

Both partners rest on the balls of their feet.
Similar to Let Us Pray (54); the man is between
his lover's legs. She places her arms around his
neck for better support and he guides her in with
his hands on her waist.

54

Let Us Pray

Both partners are on their knees, sitting back on
their legs, facing one another. He is between her
legs and can hold her for better control.

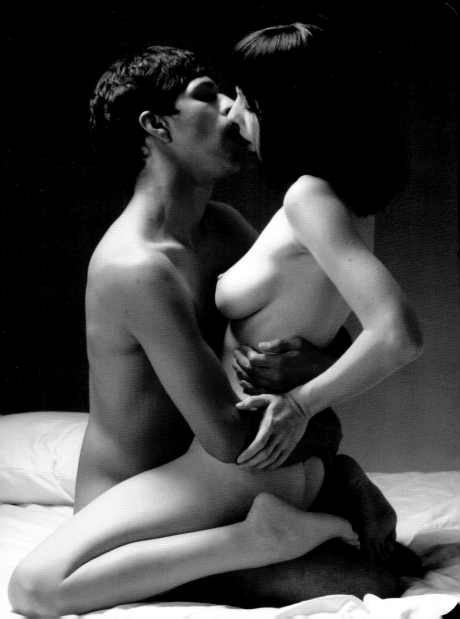

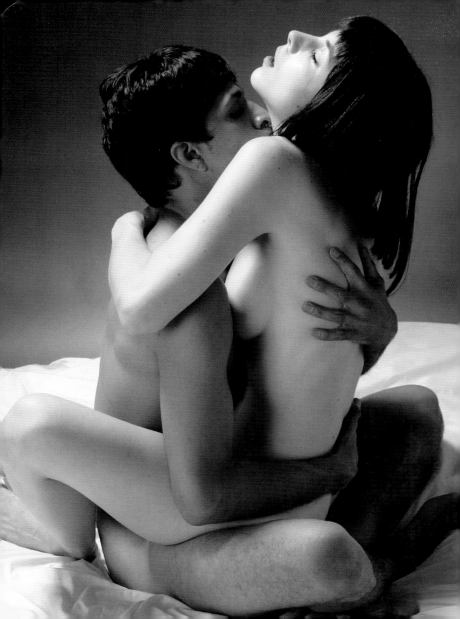

55

The Body Hug

A sitting position, where the man sits cross-legged and his partner sits in his lap facing him. She straddles him and wraps her legs around his back. This position allows the bodies to rub against each other fully and sensually.

56

Flexed Body Hug

While in the Body Hug (55), the woman raises her leg, and hangs it over her lover's arm. This alters the angle of penetration and tension between the vagina and penis.

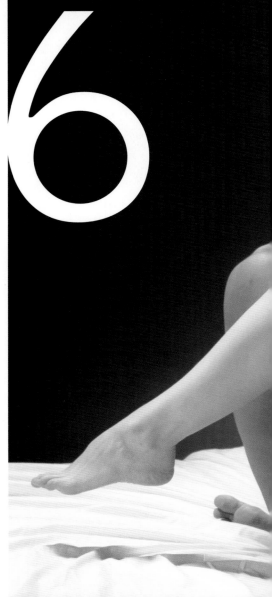

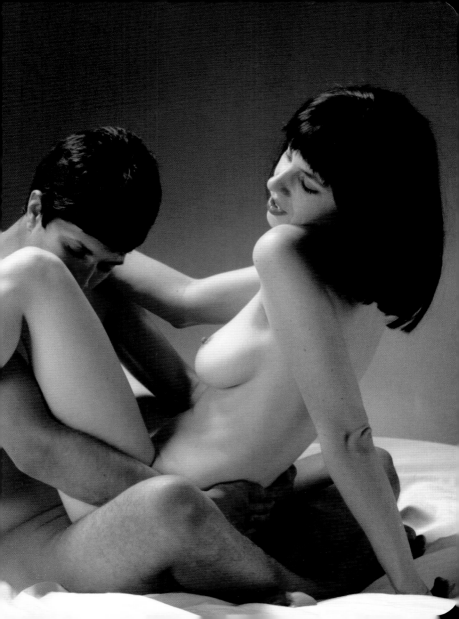

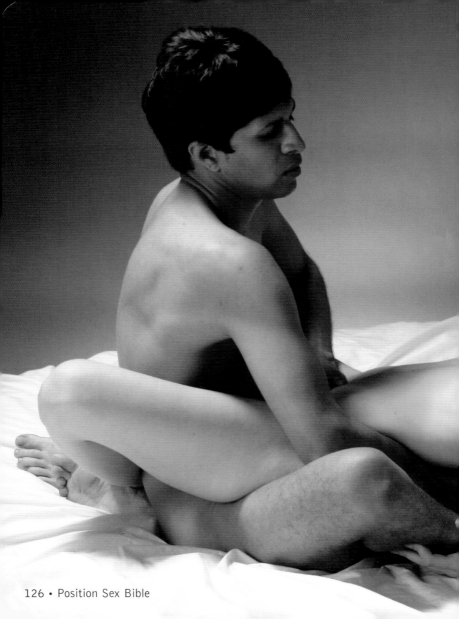

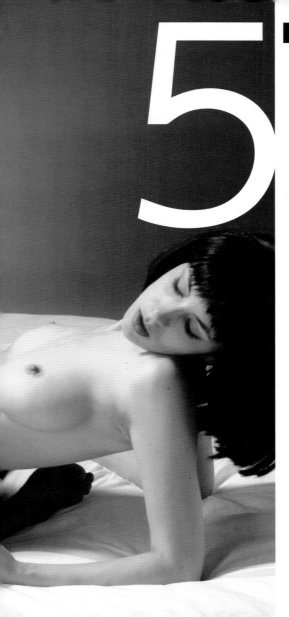

57

Reclining Body Hug

While in the Body Hug (55), the woman leans back onto her elbows, changing the angle of penetration and exposing her breasts for fondling.

58

Crying Out

From Paired Feet (39), the man slips his arms under his partner's knees and puts his hands on her waist to lift her. If there is too much strain on him, the woman can lean back and support some of her weight on her arms. The man then raises her and moves her from left to right to intensify the experience.

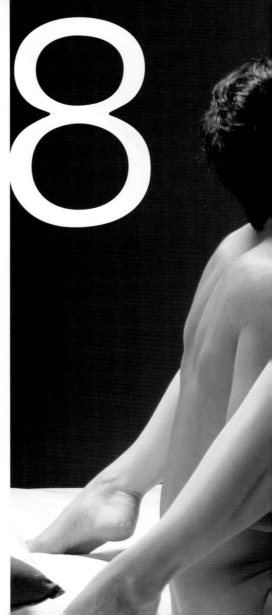

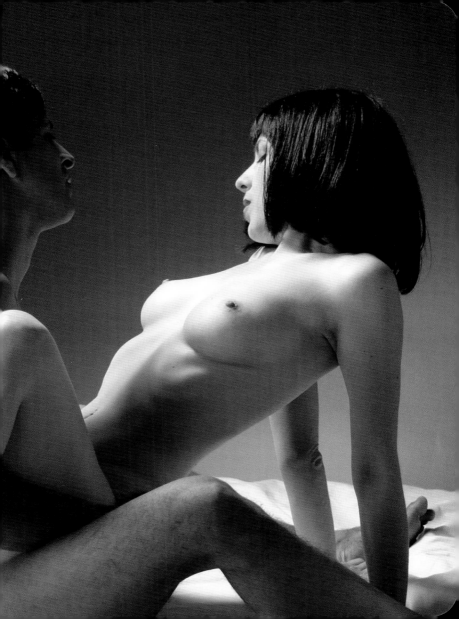

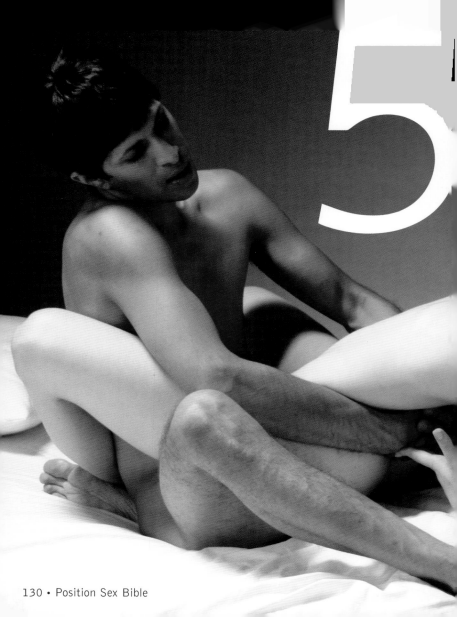

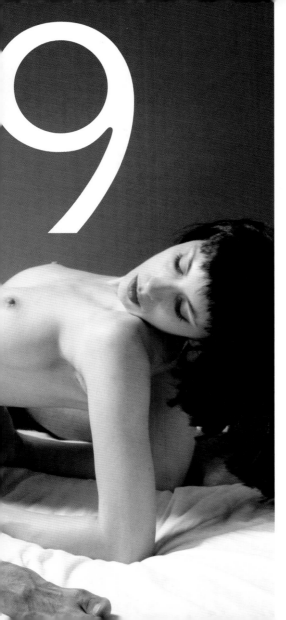

9

Sweet Abandon

The woman leans back onto her elbows, with her legs clasped behind her lover as she sits facing him.

60

The Corkscrew

While sitting up with his legs apart, knees bent and hands behind his back, the man welcomes his partner, who sits on his penis with her legs wrapped around his waist.

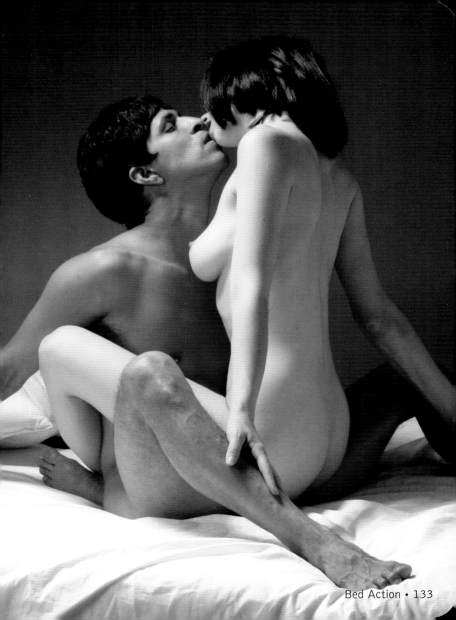

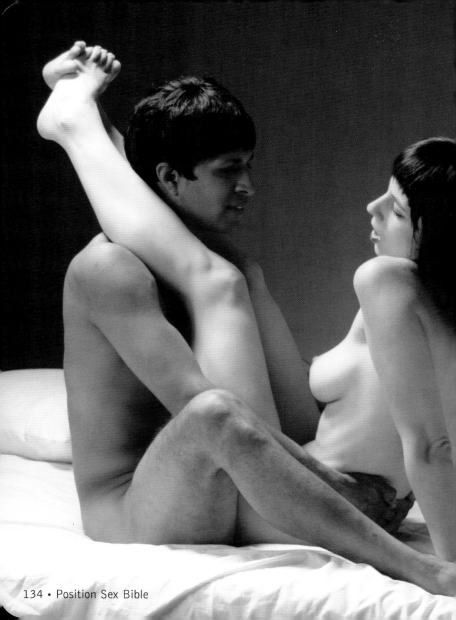

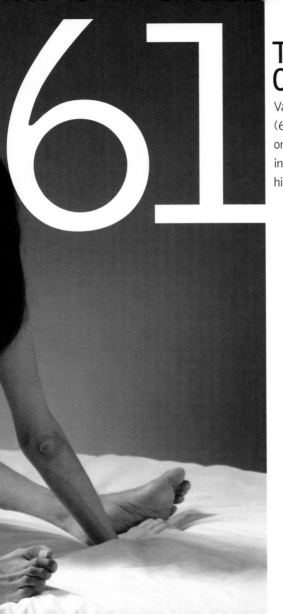

The Flexed Corkscrew

Variation on the Corkscrew (60); the woman's legs rest on her partner's shoulders instead of wrapping around his waist.

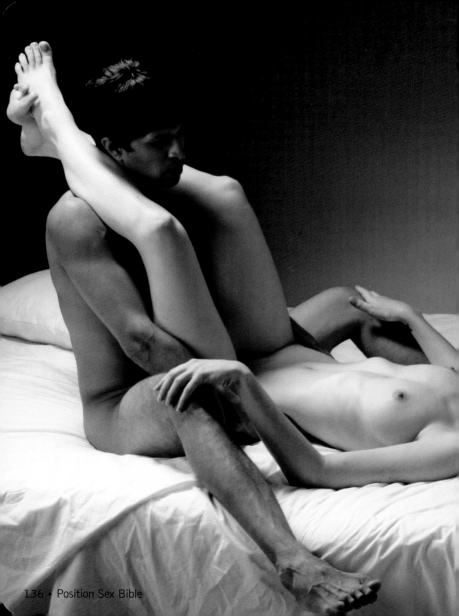

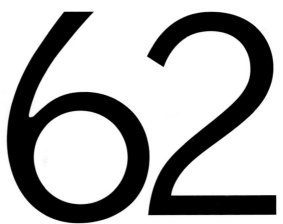

62

Inverted Headlock

The woman, on her back, faces her lover, who sits up while he straddles her. She raises her legs to either side of his head and locks her ankles behind his neck.

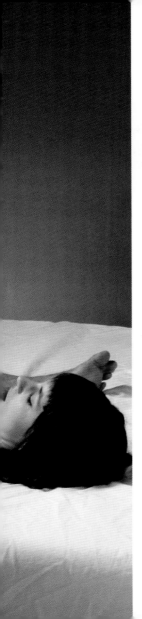

63

The See-Saw A

The man kneels and leans back on his legs, putting his arms behind him. His lover straddles him and rests her weight on the balls of her feet. She then rocks back and forth while on top.

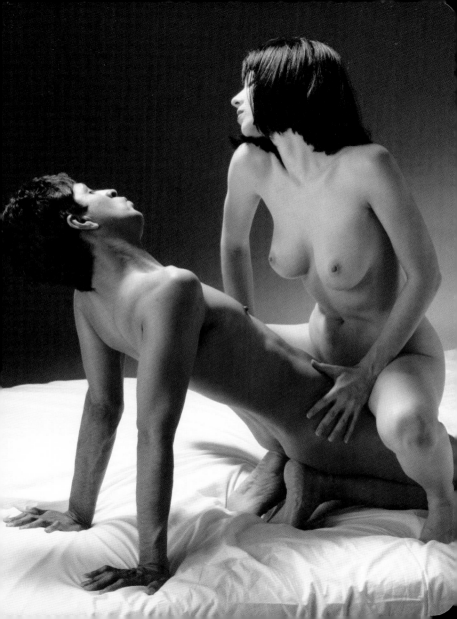

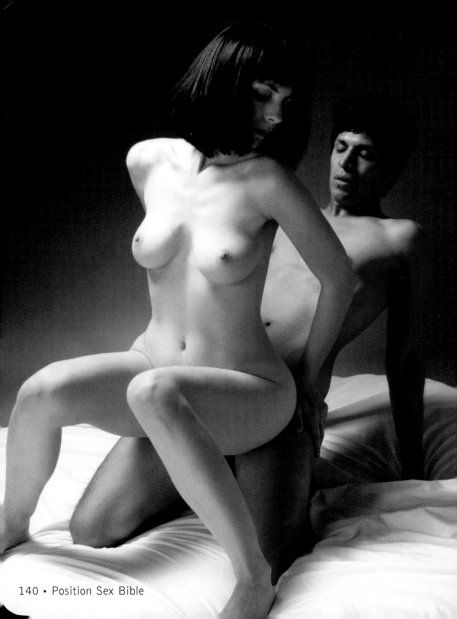

64

The See-Saw B

While in See-Saw A (63), the woman turns from facing her lover and continues with her back to him.

65

The Backbend A

Also called the Swing, the man does a backbend and maintains this position while the woman mounts and rides him.

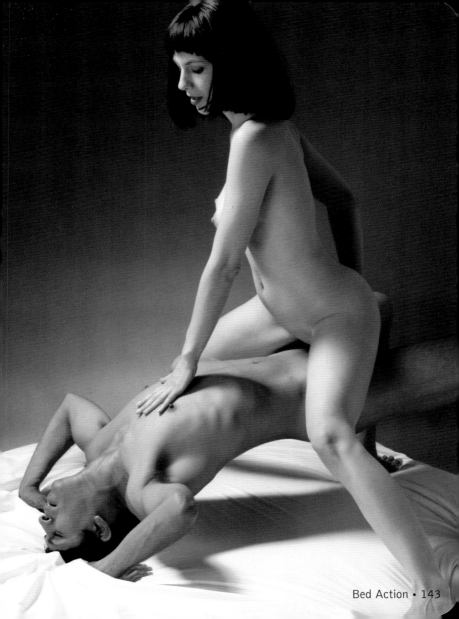

66

The Throne

The man lies back on the bed or on the
floor and bends his knees above him.
His partner sits on the back of his thighs,
which form a sort of throne, and she
mounts him in this fashion. Difficult to
maintain, but worth the effort!

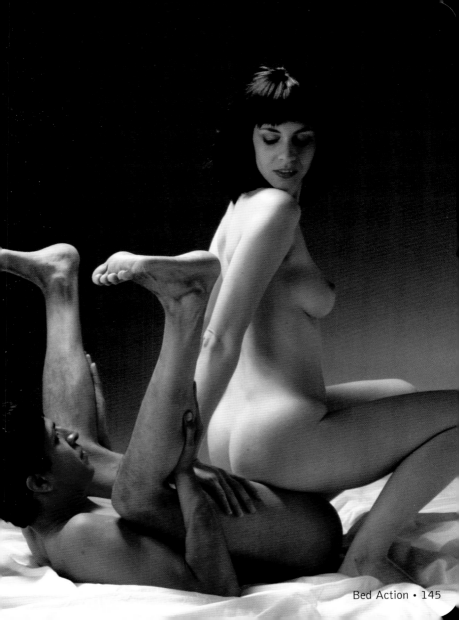

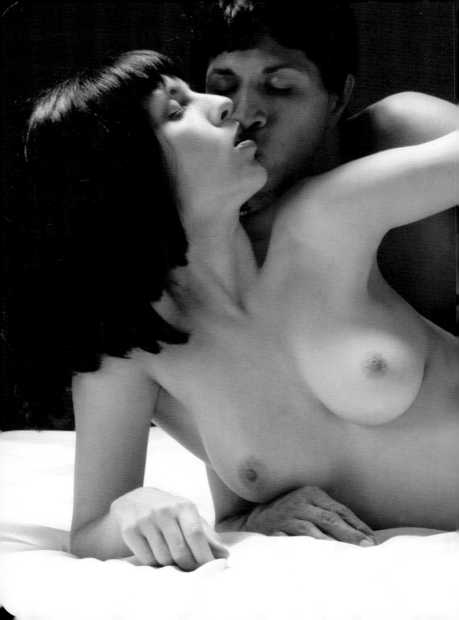

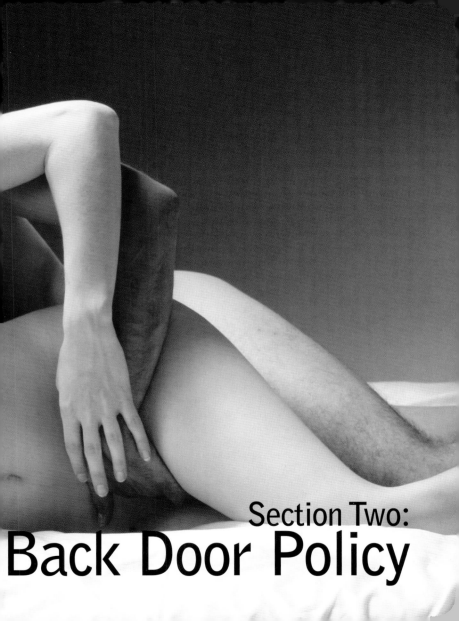

Section Two:
Back Door Policy

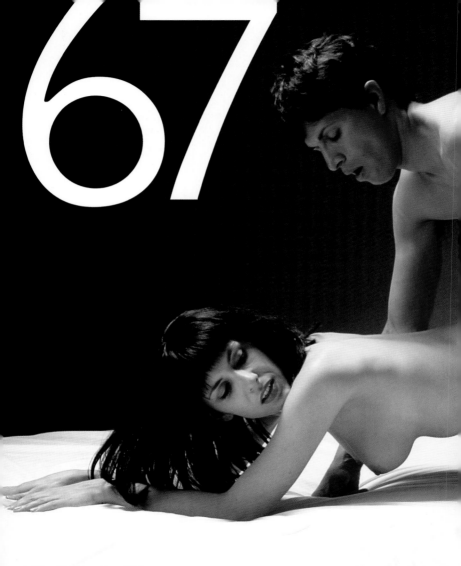

67

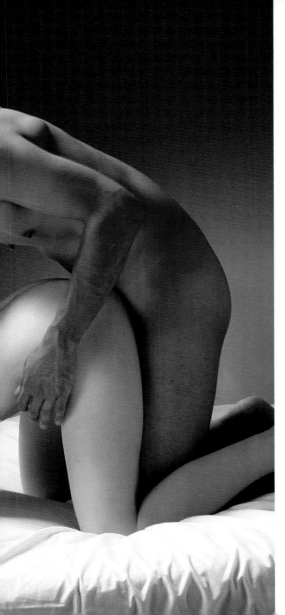

See Spot Come

The perennial doggy-style. The woman kneels on all fours and her partner kneels upright behind her, thrusting from that position. Her legs straddle his. This position allows for maximum G-spot activation.

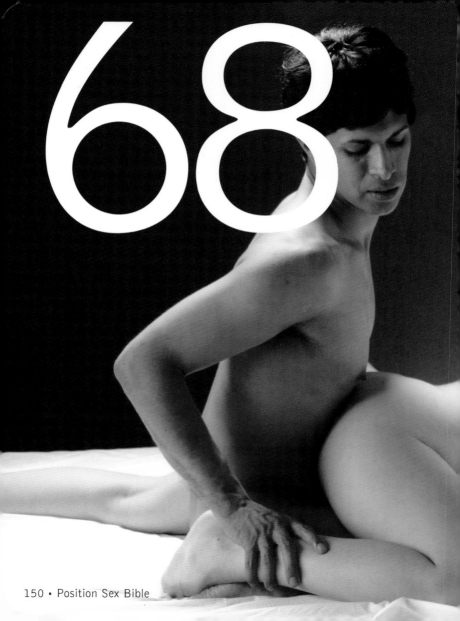

68

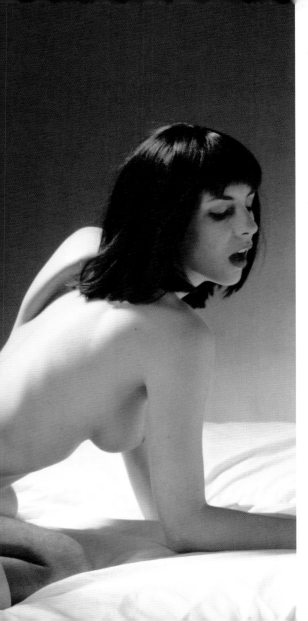

The Dutch Doggy

Variation of See Spot Come (67); requires athleticism and some well-placed pillows. The woman, while being penetrated from behind, stretches out one leg, then the other in a wind-mill motion under her lover. This position allows for intense angles of penetration.

69

Taking Sides

Variation of See Spot Come (67) that allows the man to sit instead of kneel. The woman reclines with her back to her lover, partially resting on her side and supporting herself with her elbow. (A large pillow or cushion also helps to support her body). In this position, the woman does all of the work, sliding her pelvis back and forth to intensify the experience.

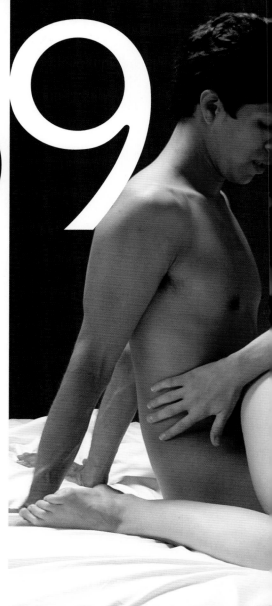

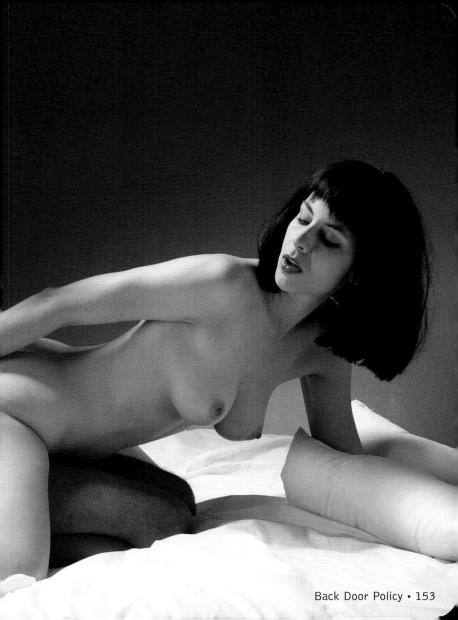

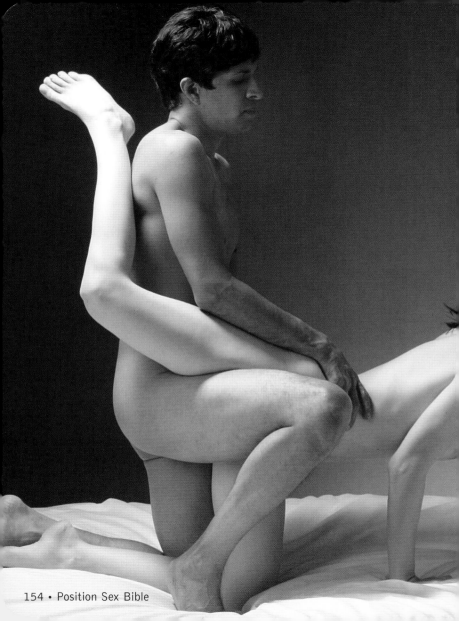

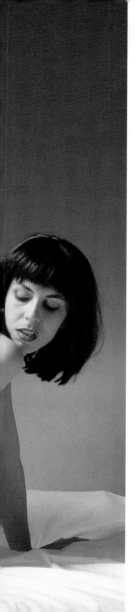

70

The Back Scratcher

The woman kneels on all fours in front of her lover,
he kneels behind her and enters her from behind.
She lifts a leg up and scratches his back with her foot.

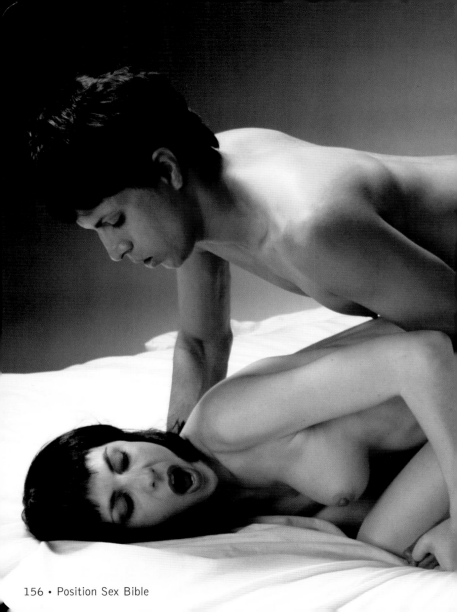

71

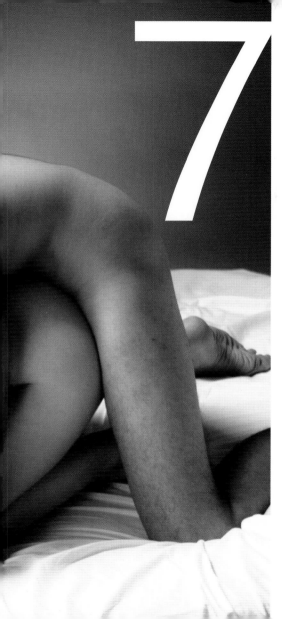

Enveloped in Love

In an inverted Press (20), the woman lies on her stomach with her legs tucked under her and the man kneels over her, entering her from behind. Her exposed back is a sensitive area that will welcome the man's gentle caresses and warm chest.

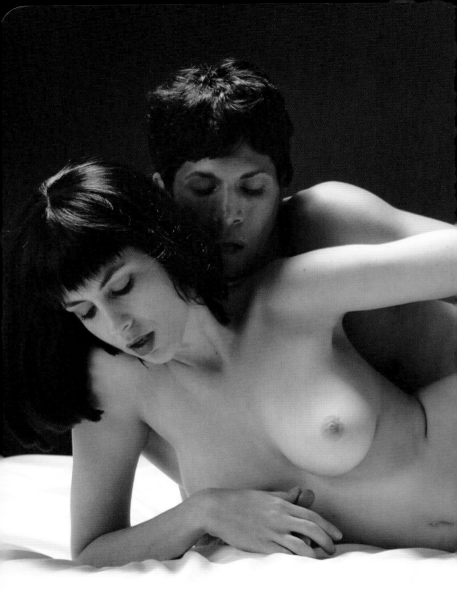

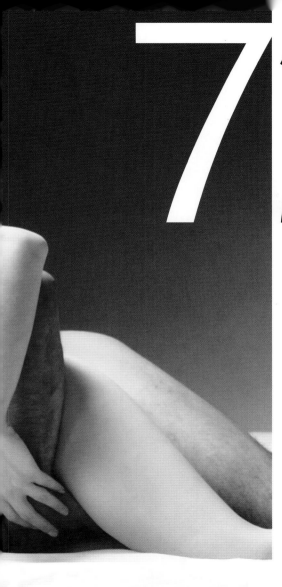

72

Baby Elephant

Prelude to the Elephant (74); both partners are on their sides, supporting themselves with one arm. The man is stretched fully behind the woman and penetrates her from this position, which frees up his other hands for breast and clitoral stimulation.

Open Elephant

While in the Baby Elephant (72), the woman opens her leg, allowing for better clitoral stimulation.

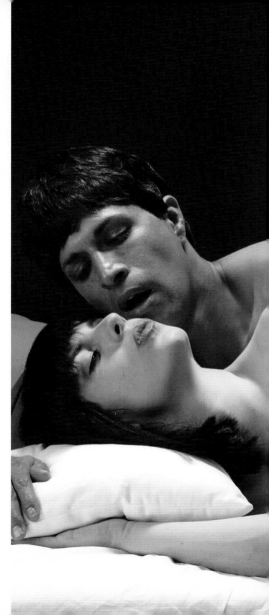

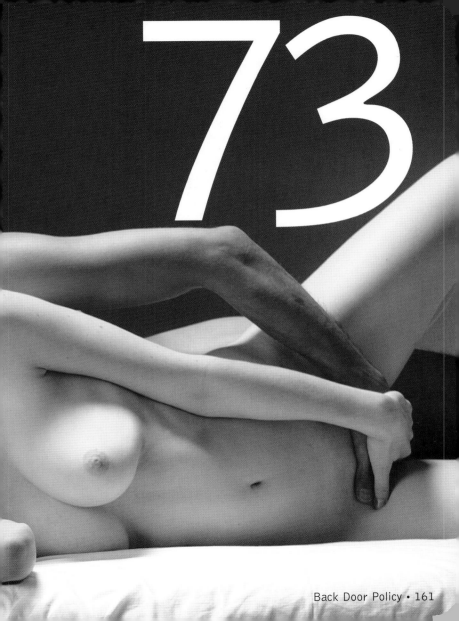

73

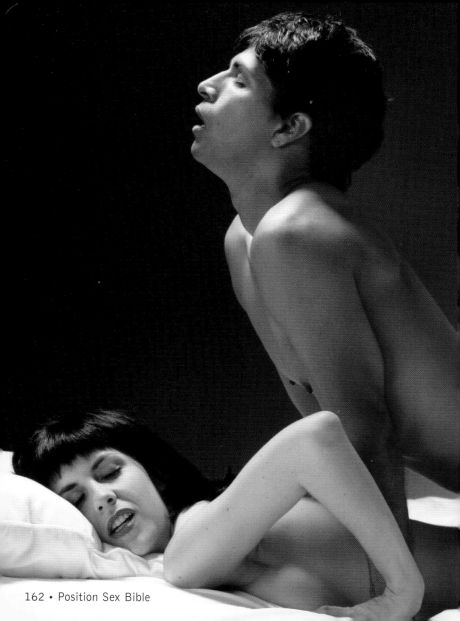

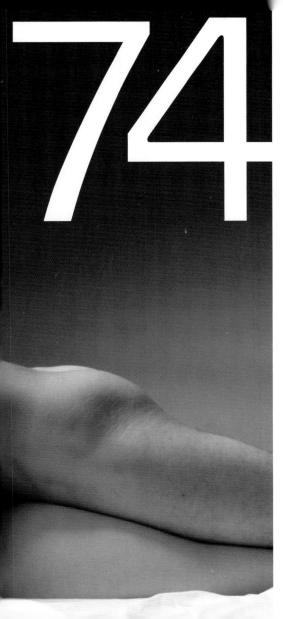

74

The Elephant

The woman lies on her stomach and the man lies on top of her, full body. His legs lie straight between hers and he penetrates her from behind, forgoing kissing and eye contact, but increasing G-spot activation angles and deep penetration.

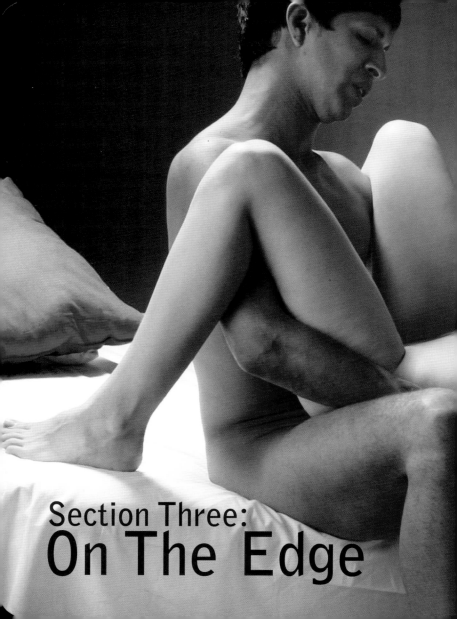

Section Three:
On The Edge

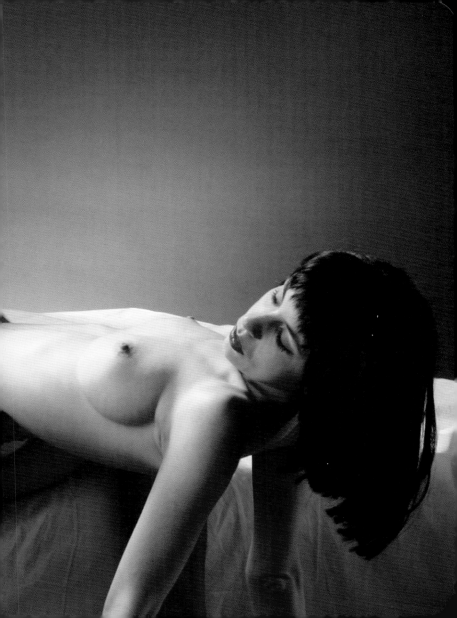

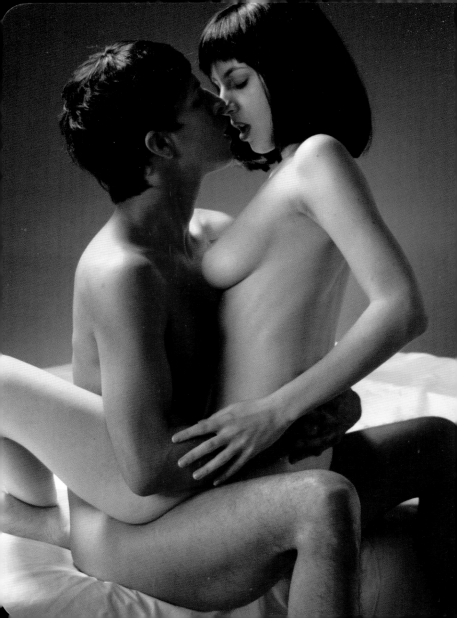

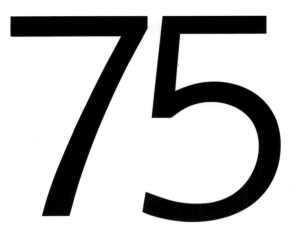

Sitting Body Wrap

The man sits on the edge of the bed or in a backless chair; his partner sits on his lap facing him and wraps her legs around his back.

76

Sitting Flexed Body Wrap

While in the Sitting Body Wrap (75), the woman hangs her legs over her lover's arms, allowing for even closer contact and better clitoral stimulation.

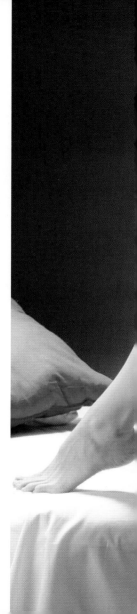

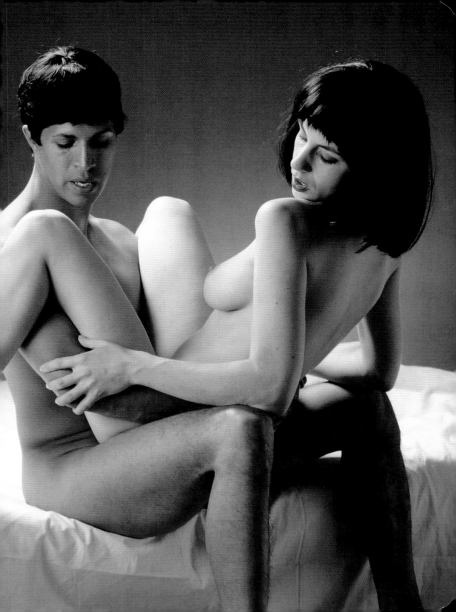

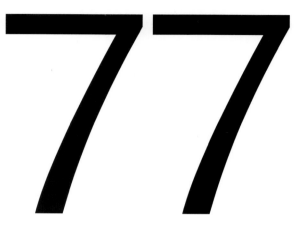

The Backbend B

While in the Sitting Body Wrap (75), the woman does a backbend, easing her hands behind her so that her palms rest on the floor.

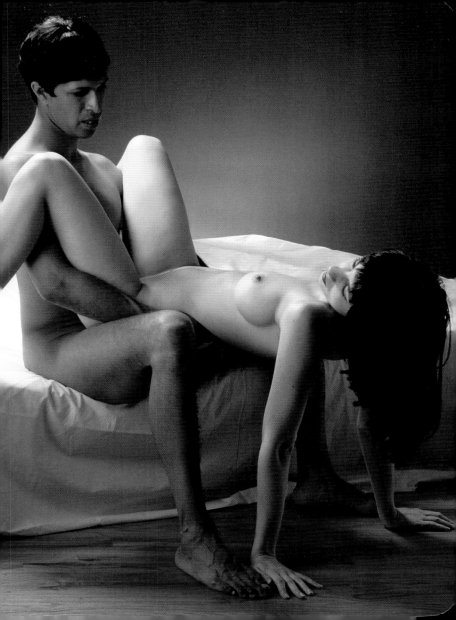

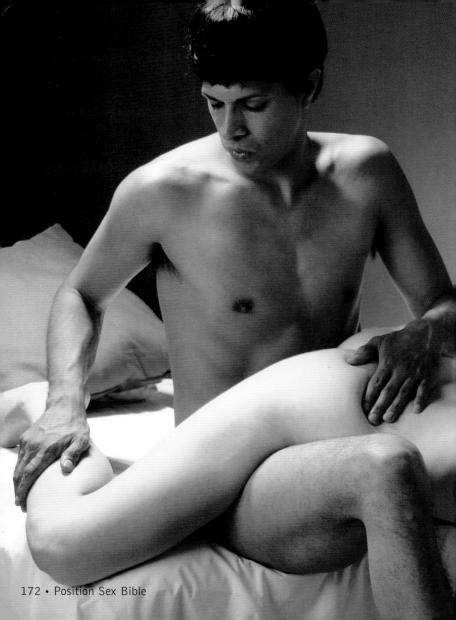

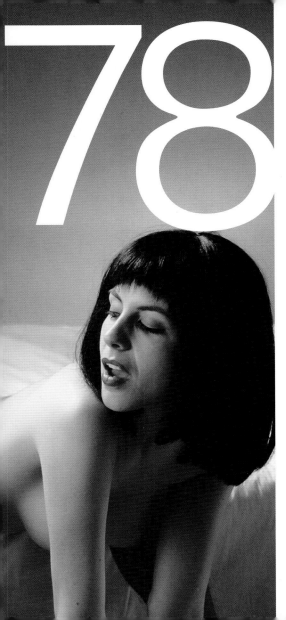

78

The Pushover

The woman's legs wrap around the waist of her lover, and she leans forward over his lap and places her hands on the floor. Perfect prelude to the Hoover (87).

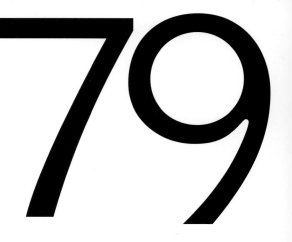

The Cobra

From the Pushover (78), the woman raises her
torso and rests her hands on the knees of her
seated lover.

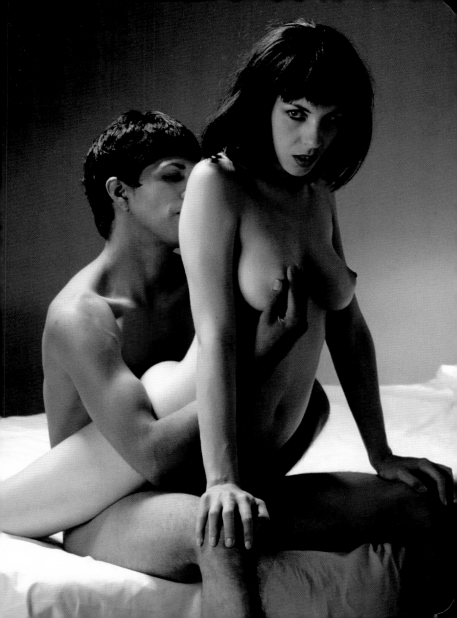

80

The Pilot

Instead of being a Pushover (78), the woman extends her legs back and her arms to her sides, assuming an airplane position while on her lover's lap.

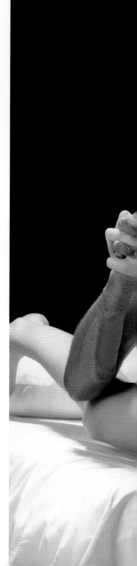

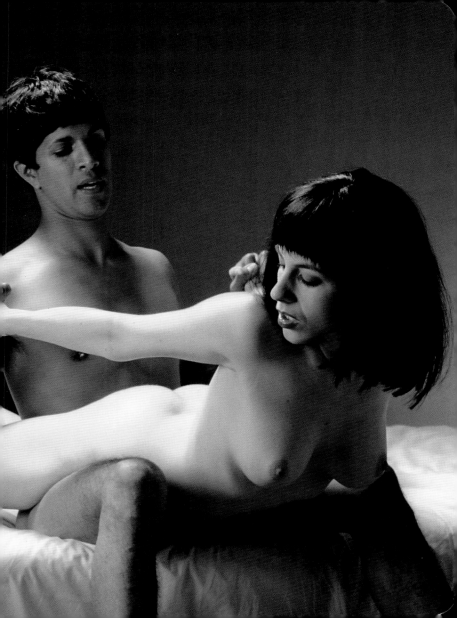

Section Four:
The Standing O

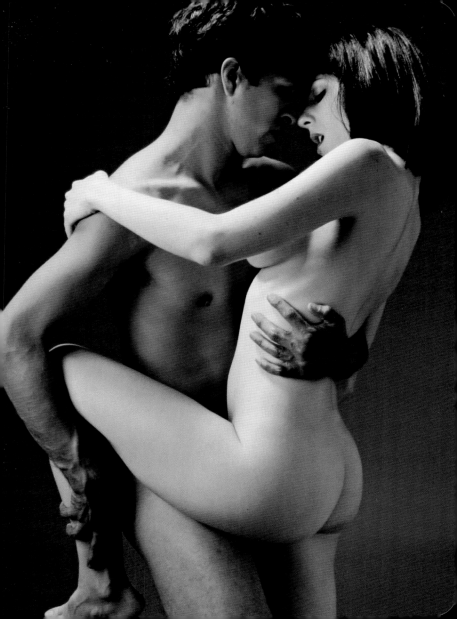

81

The Stick Up

From the Tango (83), the woman turns to have her back to her lover and lifts one knee up, which the man can hold in place. He then has access to enter her from behind.

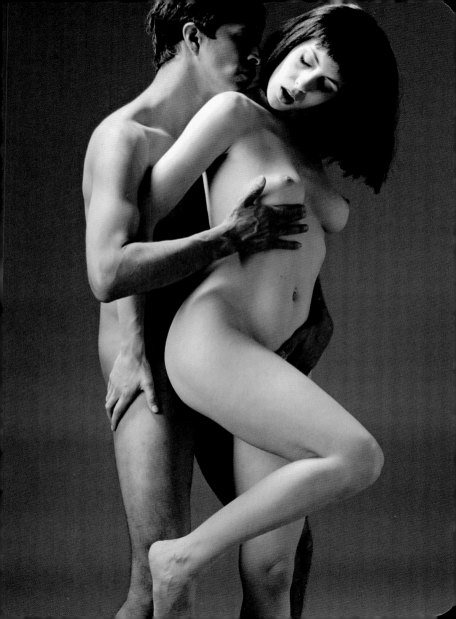

82

Stand by Your Man

The woman stands in front of her lover with her back to him. She straddles him, bending one leg behind his back. She may need to hold onto him for balance.

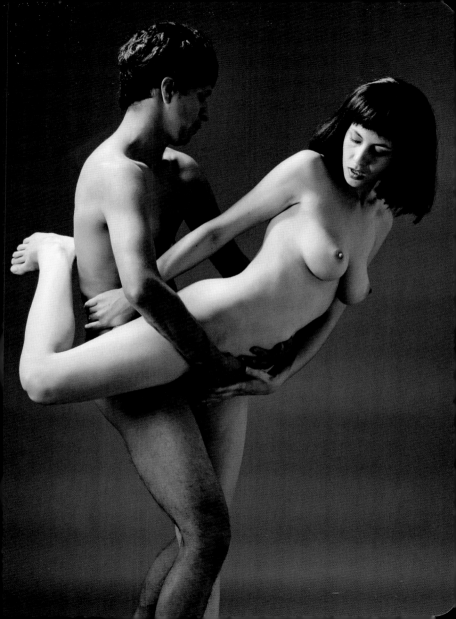

83

The Tango

Both partners stand and face each other.
The woman wraps her arms around her lover's
neck and one leg around his for leverage.

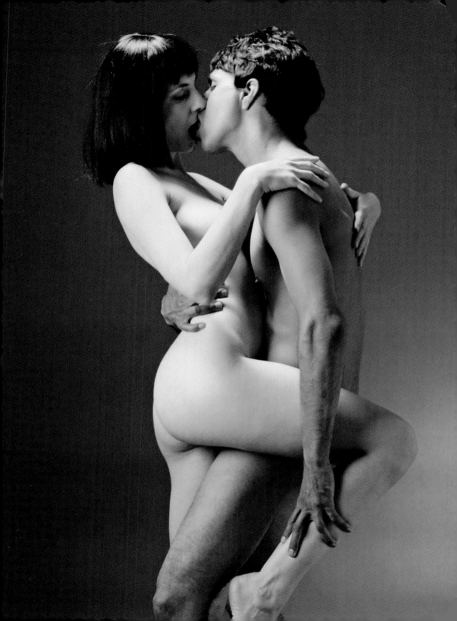

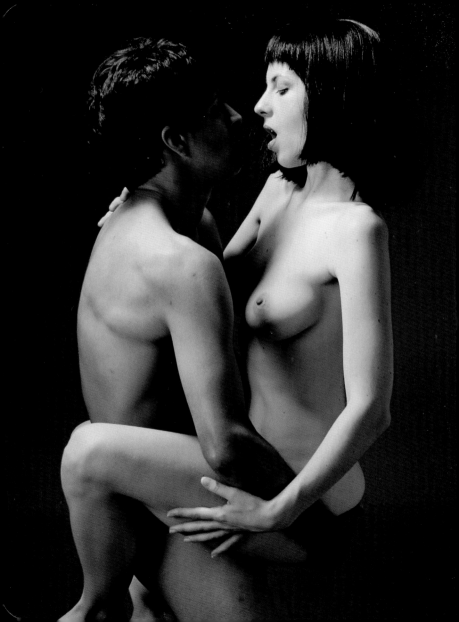

84

The Harness

The man stands with his feet shoulder-width apart. He holds his partner as she wraps her legs around his waist. This position requires strong upper-body strength for the man.

85

The Backbend C

While in the Harness (84), the woman eases herself back and tries to touch the floor with her hands. Her legs are still locked behind her lover's back for control and his arms must be strong to support her weight. To reduce the strain on both partners, try it off of the bed instead.

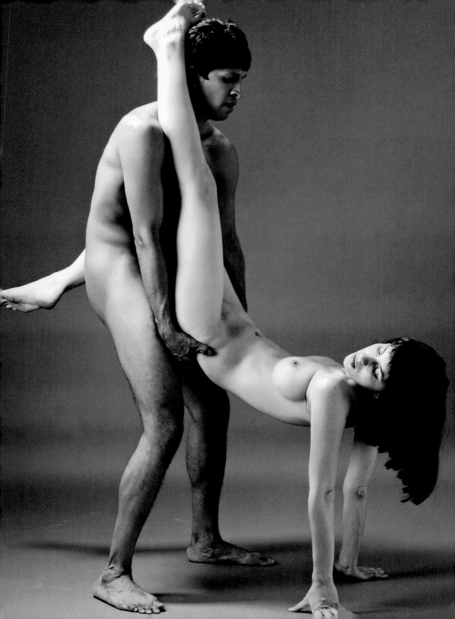

86

Congress of the Cow

The woman stands on the ground and places her palms flat in front of her, (or on the bed or a chair if she is not flexible enough). The man enters her from behind, and has full access to her buttocks in this powerful sexual stance. If the woman begins to feels lightheaded, move into the Stick Up (81).

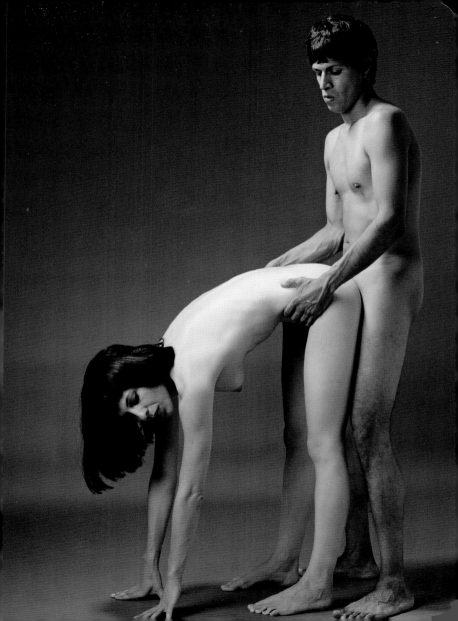

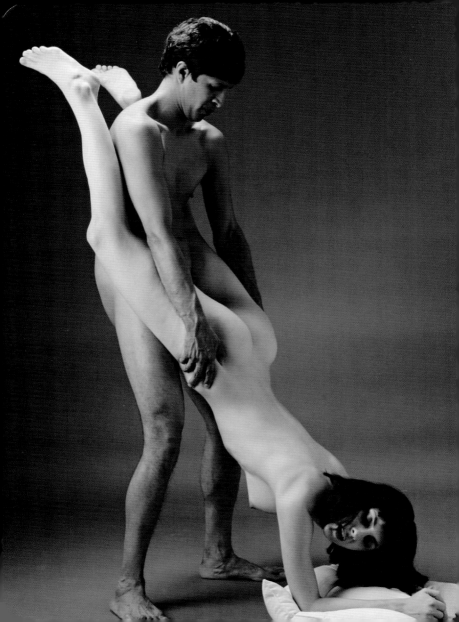

87

The Hoover

The woman rests her forearms on the floor while her partner lifts the rest of her body waist-level and enters her from behind. She can clasp her legs around her lover's waist for better control.

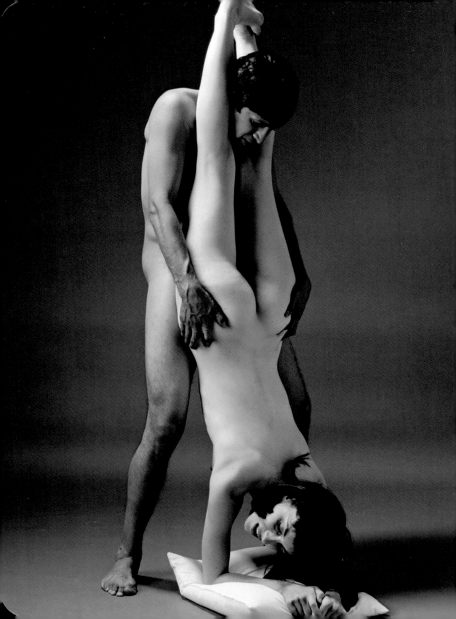

88

The Hoover Upright

The Hoover (87), but with the woman's feet
clasped behind her lover's neck.

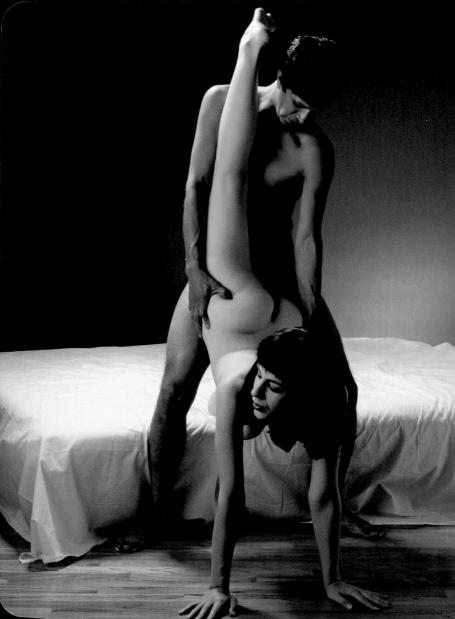

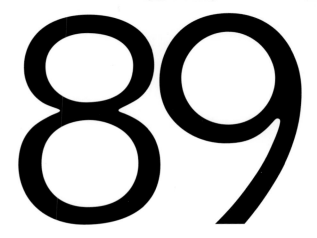

The Handstand

The Hoover Upright (88), but a little higher.
The woman shifts her weight to her palms instead
of resting on her forearms.

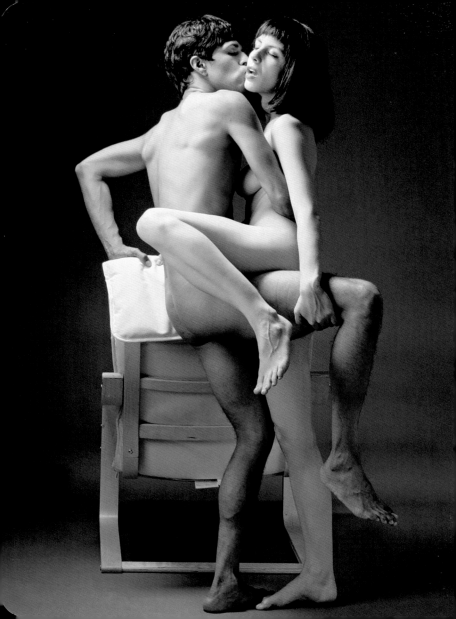

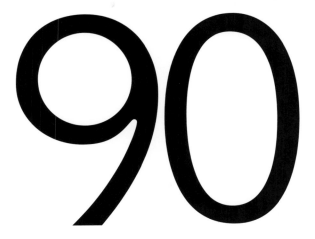

The Leg Up

Both lovers face each other while standing.
The woman drapes her left leg over her partner's
thigh and grabs on to allow for deep penetration.

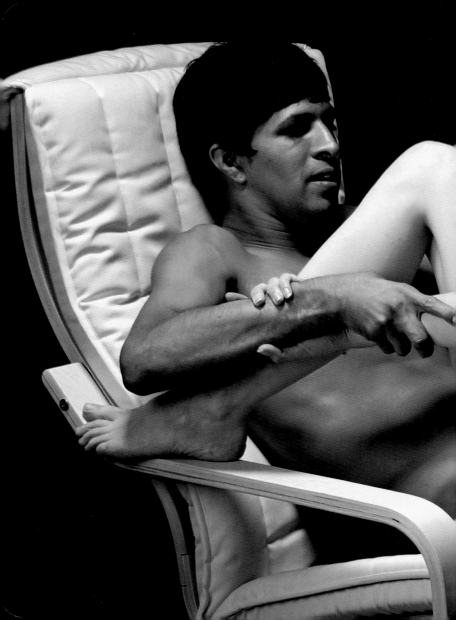

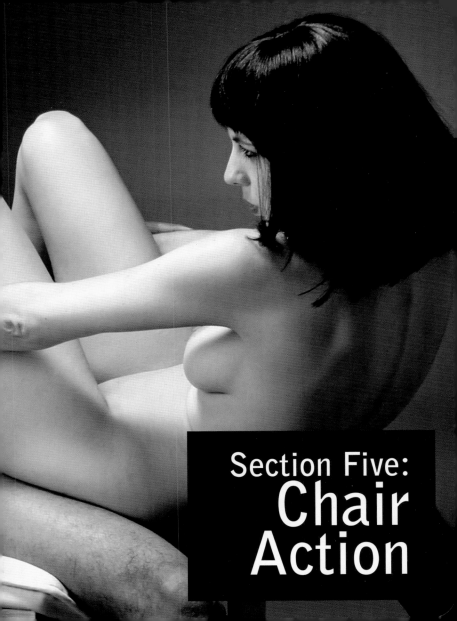

Section Five:
Chair
Action

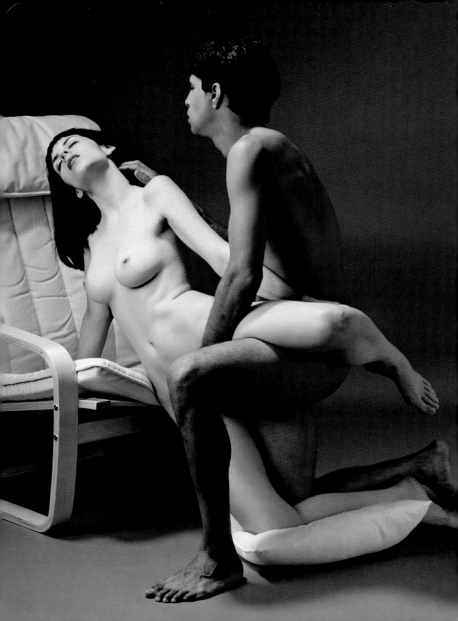

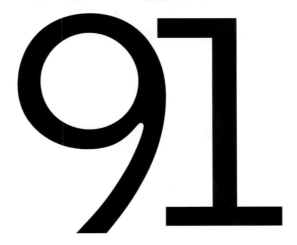

The Chair Lift

With the help of a chair and a cushion, this kneeling position allows for deep penetration and new angles. The woman leans on the chair sideways, while her lover kneels in front of her. She can drape a leg over his thigh, allowing for clitoral stimulation.

92

Purrfect Plunge

The Cat position; similar to See Spot Come (67)
without the woman as prostrate. The woman kneels
upright and leans over a bed or rests against
a chair while her lover enters her from behind. The
woman's legs remain in between his, and her
vertical posture allows for the fondling of her
breasts and clitoris.

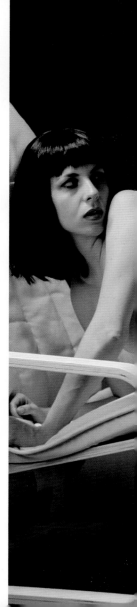

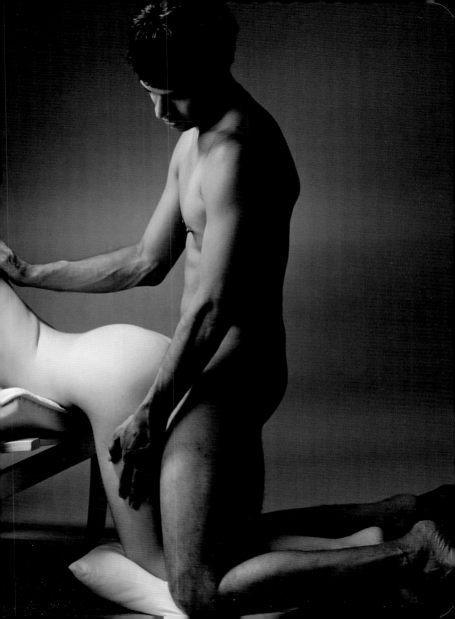

93

The Lounge Cat

While assuming the Purrfect Plunge
(92) on a chair, the woman is ready
for her lover to stand and enter her
from behind.

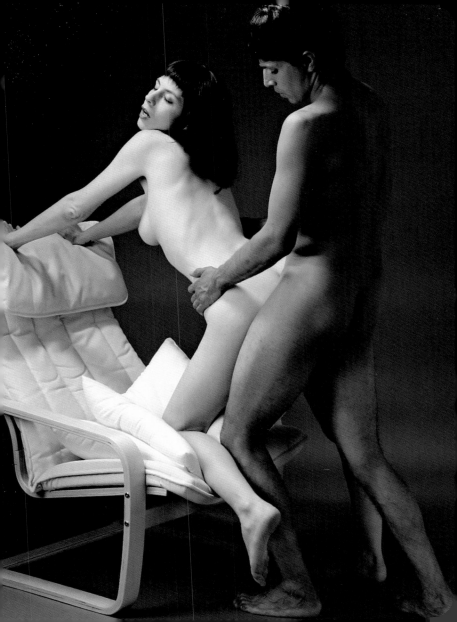

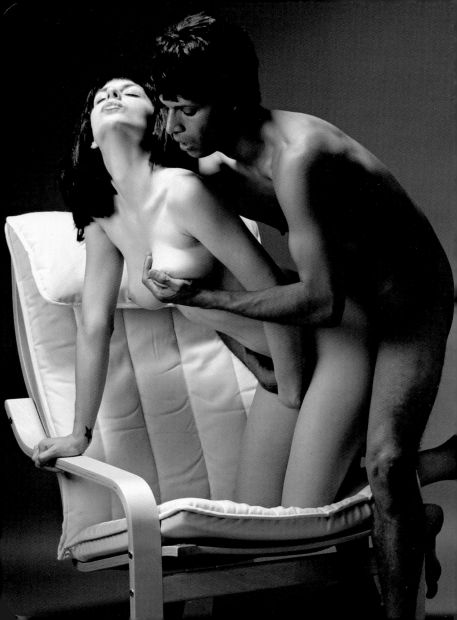

94

Fido's on His Feet

Doggy-style off the bed. The woman is on all fours or simply kneeling on a chair, and the man stands behind her, mounting her from this position.

95

The Wheelbarrow

The Hoover (87) for your bed or chair.
Same concept, except that the woman has a
cushiony support for her forearms, and the
angle is not as extreme.

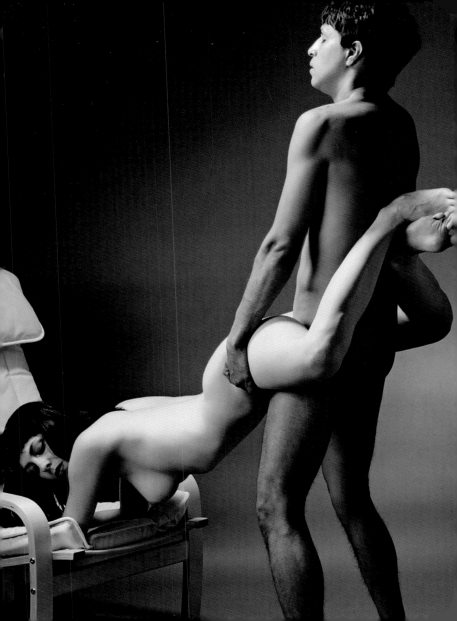

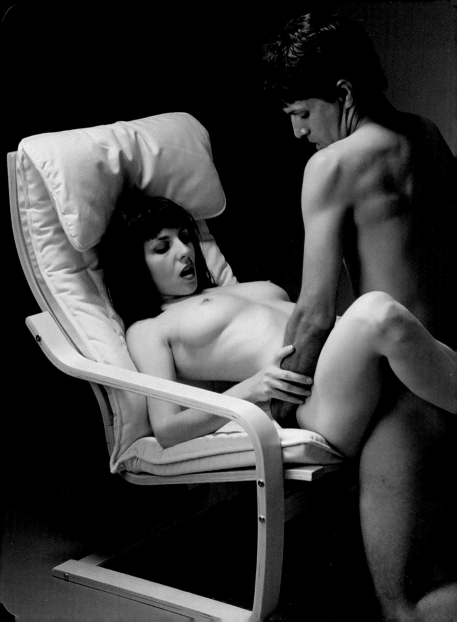

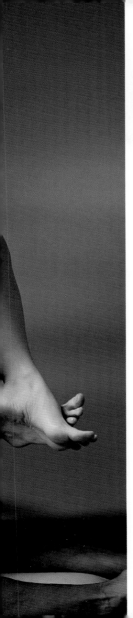

96

Lay-Z Girl

The woman sits in a large easy chair and the man kneels in front of her. She wraps her legs around his back. Easy on both partners, as no one has to support the other's weight.

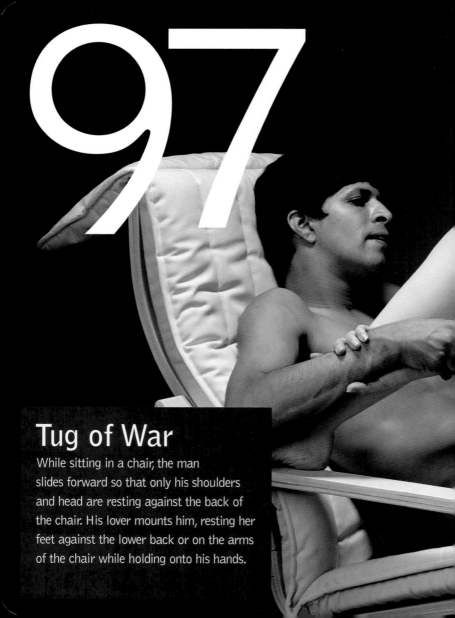

97

Tug of War

While sitting in a chair, the man slides forward so that only his shoulders and head are resting against the back of the chair. His lover mounts him, resting her feet against the lower back or on the arms of the chair while holding onto his hands.

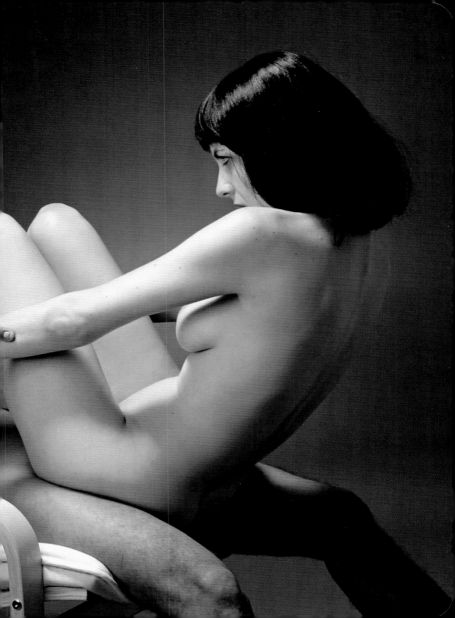

98

Come Sit on My Lap

The man sits or lies on a chair and his partner slips onto his lap backwards.

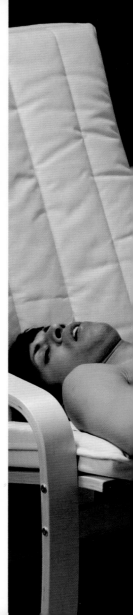

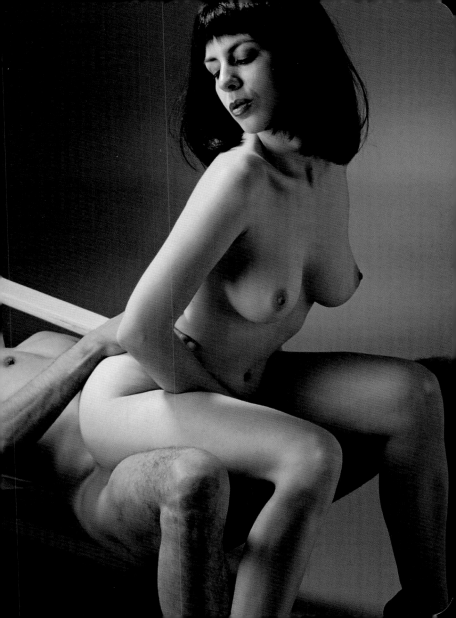

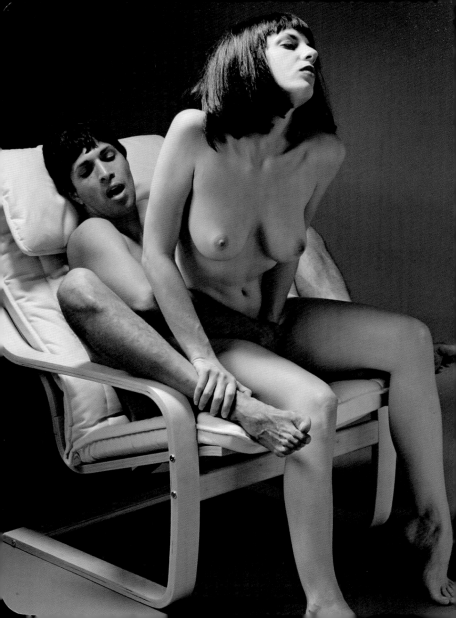

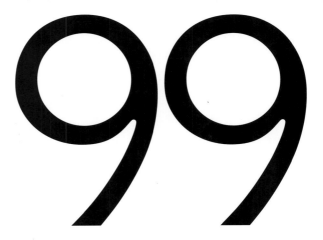

In Reverse

Instead of sitting on her lover's lap, the woman stands with her back to him while he is in the chair and holds up his legs while he enters her from behind, pulling her down onto him.

100

My Knight, My Chair

The man lies in a chair upside-down. His lover mounts him from above, resting her knees on the arms of the chair. He can hold her ankles for support, so he doesn't slip off. (He could get light-headed, so work quickly!)

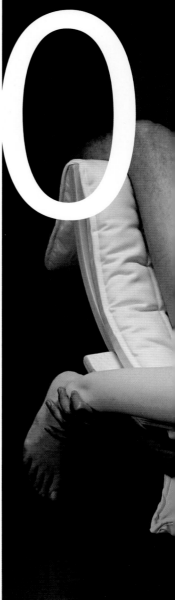

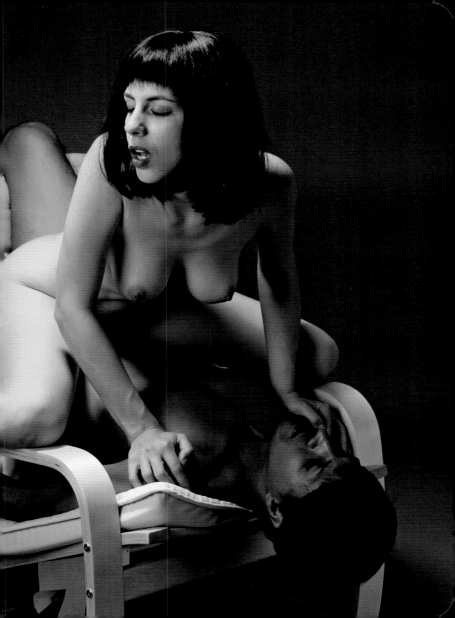

101

Chair Twister

The man sits in a chair and the woman gets in the Hoover (87) in front of him, with her legs resting on either side of his face. Both partners win, but the games have just begun!

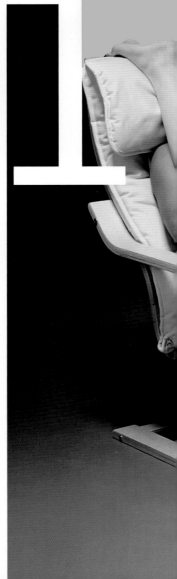

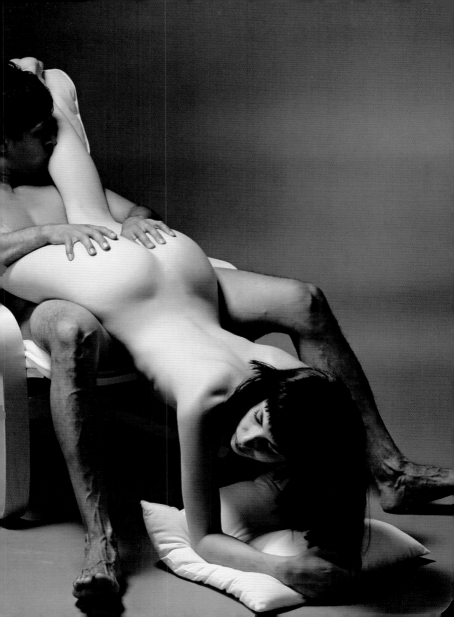

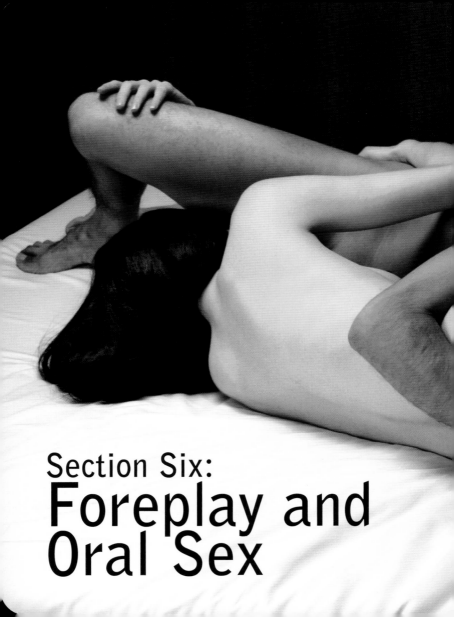

Section Six:
Foreplay and Oral Sex

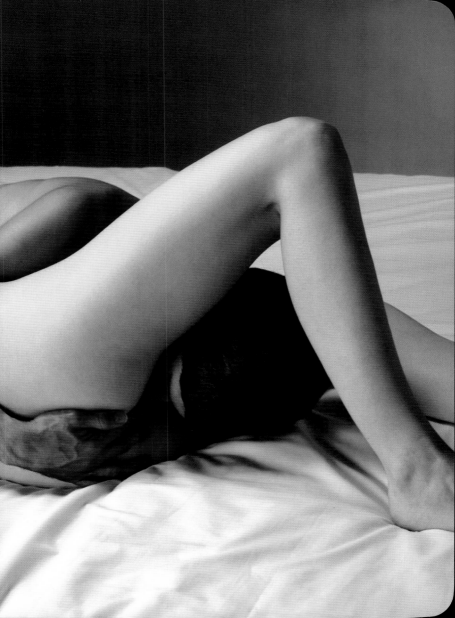

102

Backseat Driver

Both lovers face the same direction on the
bed with the man sitting between the
woman's legs and her breasts pressed
against his back. She reaches around his
torso with both hands and encircles his
penis, bringing him to orgasm while she
enjoys watching over his shoulder.

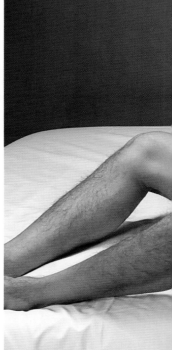

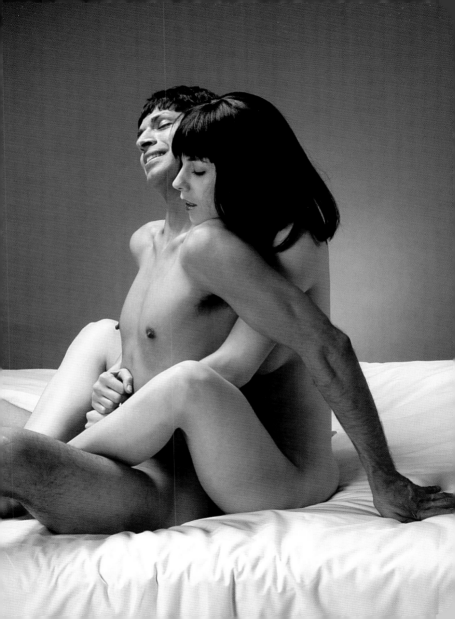

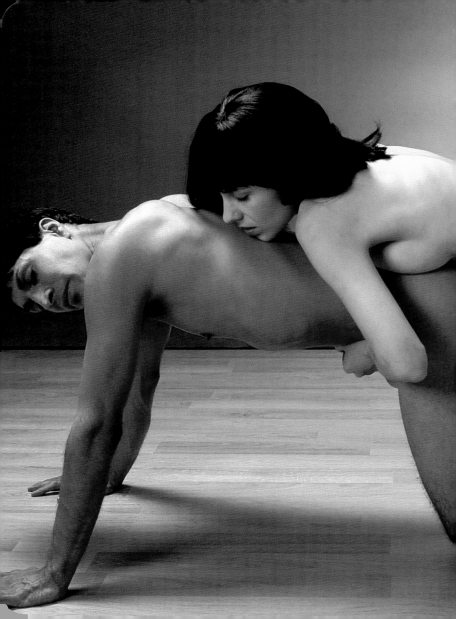

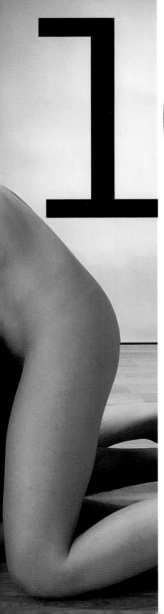

103

Prepare for Takeoff

With the man on all fours, the woman grabs him tightly from the rear with her torso flattened against his buttocks. She massages his penis with one hand and reaches between his legs with the other, fondling his testicles while he comes to climax.

104

The Magic Lamp

The woman lies on her back while the man pushes her leg high up against her body. With open access to her taut labia, the man rubs her. He maintains the contrast between the tight grip on her ankle and more fluid motion of hand on her genitals, coaxing her to orgasm.

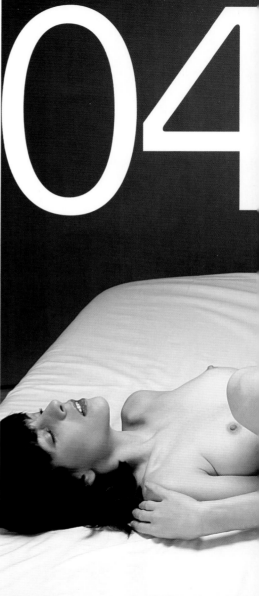

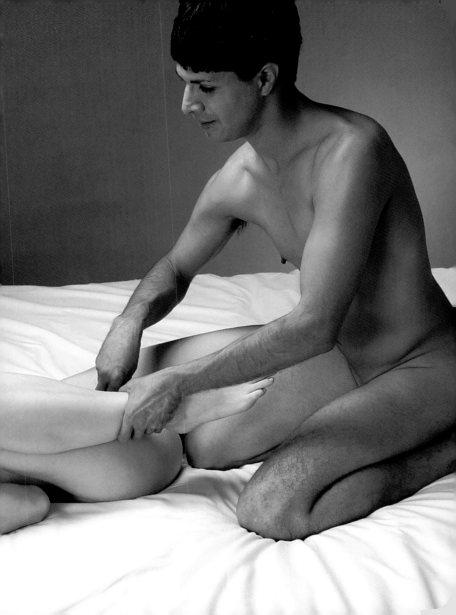

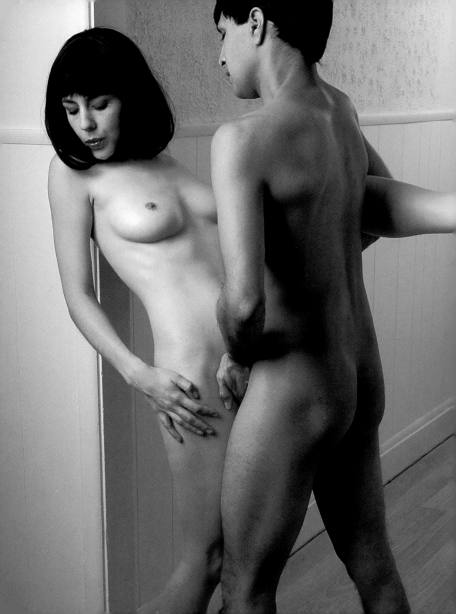

105

Third Wish

Variation of the Magic Lamp with the couple standing up, the woman's back against a wall or doorway. The man lifts her leg with one hand and "rubs her lamp" with the other.

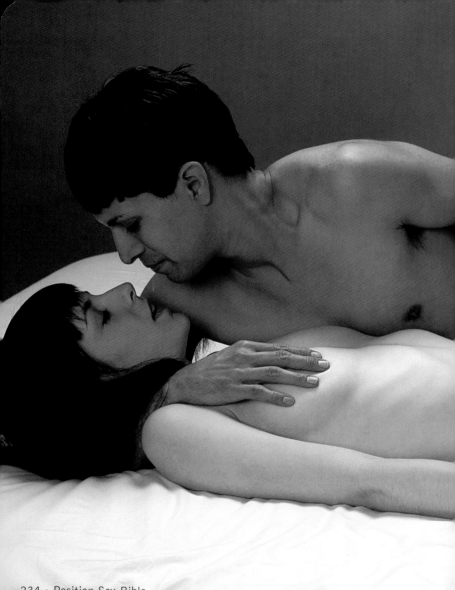

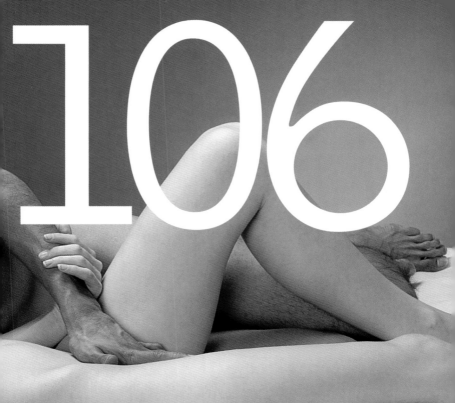

106

Cat in the Cradle

The woman lies on her back while the man lies on his side next to her. One arm slips under her neck and reaches down to fondle her breast. The other slips in between her legs massaging and teasing and eventually hooking inside her. The man kisses her, capturing her complete sensory experience.

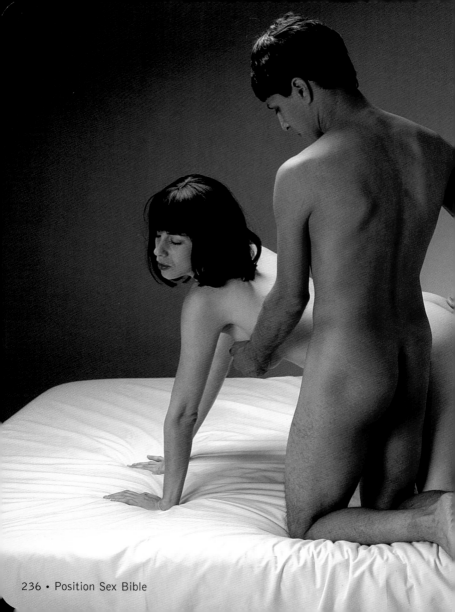

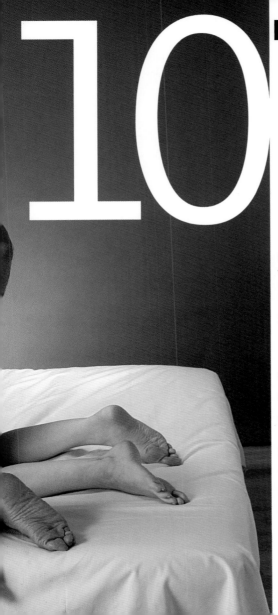

107

Spank
Her Thrice

She's on all fours.
He kneels beside her.
He caresses her breasts
while his other hand
explores her back, belly
and thighs, at last find-
ing her vagina. He grabs
her buttock, holding it
tight, and maybe gives
her a slap. This is a
good prelude to See
Spot Come (67).

108

The Double Grip

Moving from The Crab (17), he holds her feet with his thumbs between her big toes and the rest. He enters her, pressing her knees against her breasts, stimulating her vagina and feet for a double erogenous explosion.

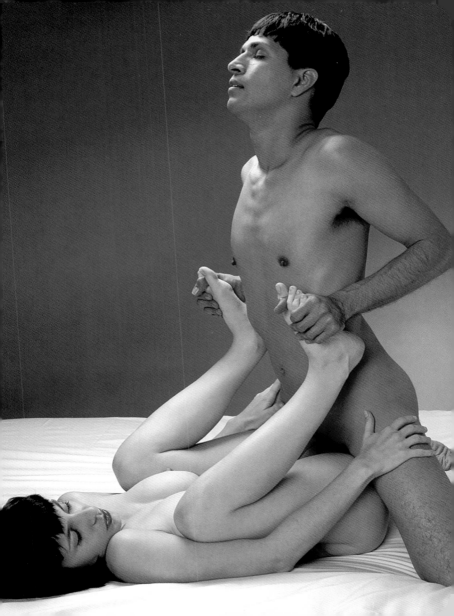

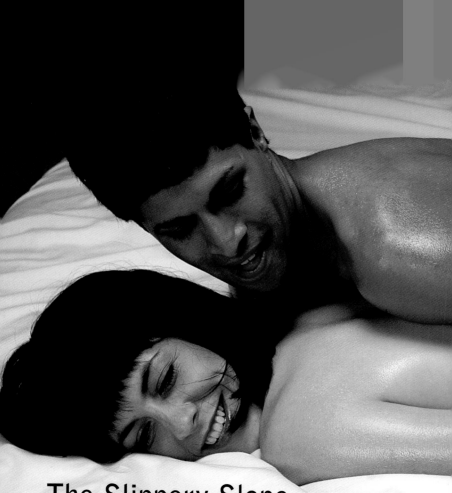

The Slippery Slope

Covered in massage oil, the man and woman take turns slipping and sliding over each other, first with her facing downward and him on top of her and then reversing. Penetration is not the goal, just sensuous stimulation.

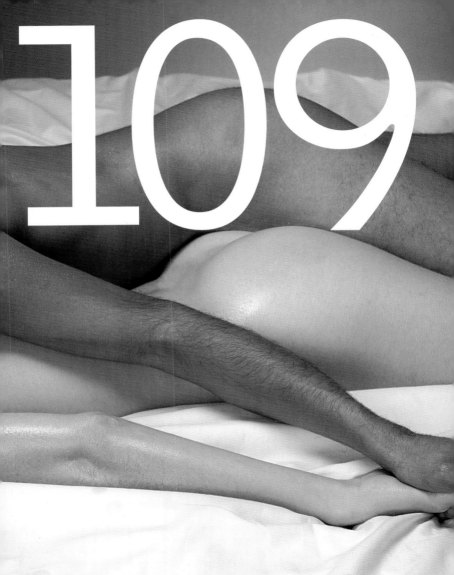

109

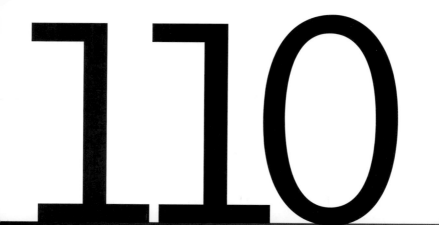

110

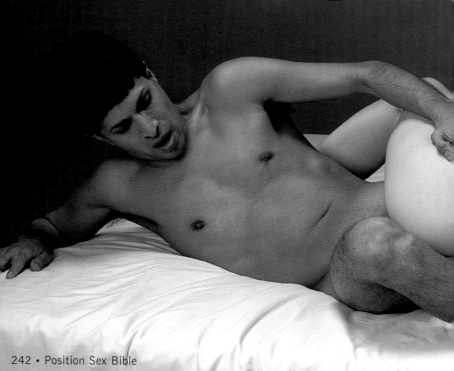

Jigsaw

The woman curls up on the bed, her delicate parts exposed to her lover. He embraces her with his legs and fits in perfectly.

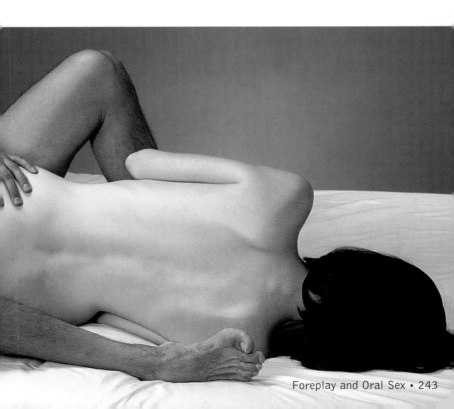

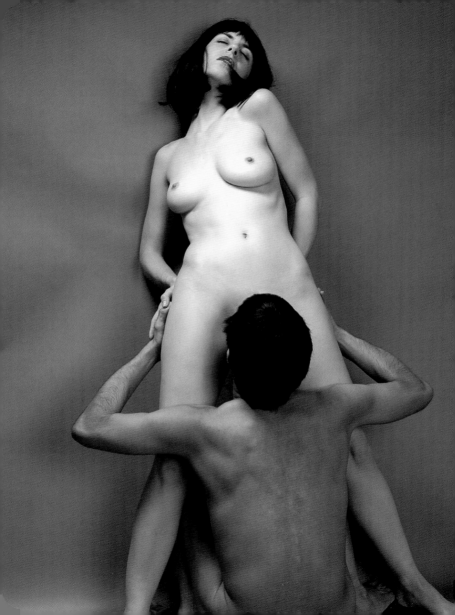

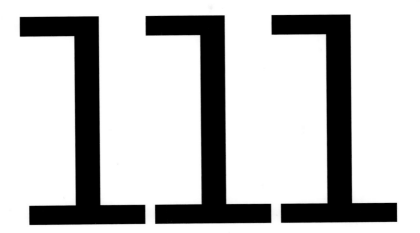

111

Put You on a Pedestal

Woman or man leans against the wall, legs spread.
Partner sits on the floor between spread legs,
wrapping arms around lower back and pays
homage to the other.

112

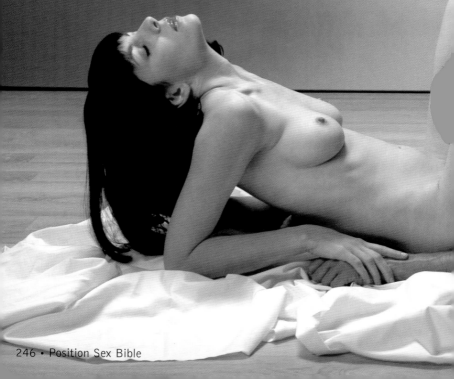

Under the Hood

Woman sits on floor leaning back on her forearms. Man kneels in front between her legs, bending down into her labia. She rests her legs on his back while he licks her.

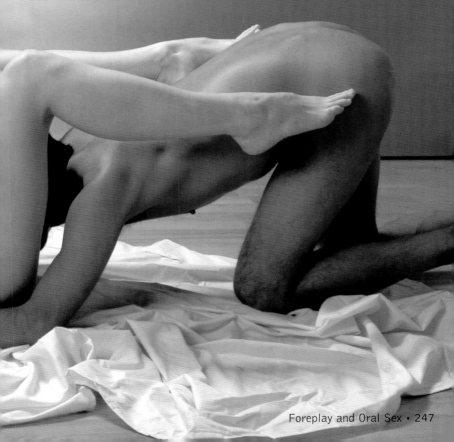

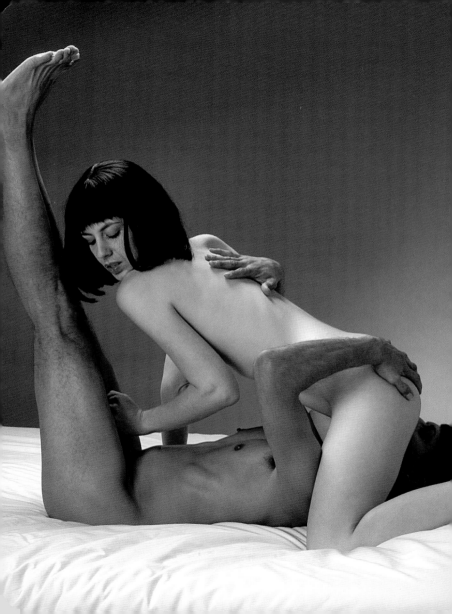

113

Pumping Petrol

Man lies on his back with his legs straight up. Woman sits on man's face, and grabs his penis, bringing him to climax while he does the same for her.

114

Sweet Spot

The couple lies head to foot. The man moves the woman's knees up and out of the way as he delves between her legs. She reaches for his penis. He covers her genitals with his mouth.

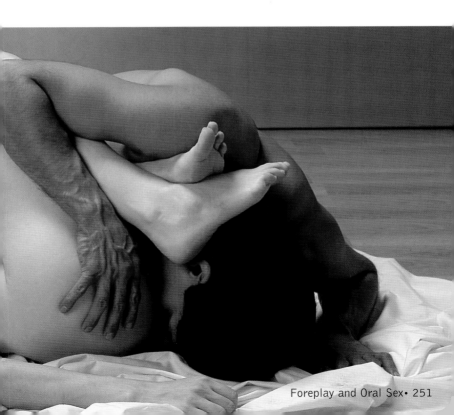

115

Australian for Sex

Woman lies on her back with her legs in the air.
Man lies on his stomach with his head down under,
between her legs.

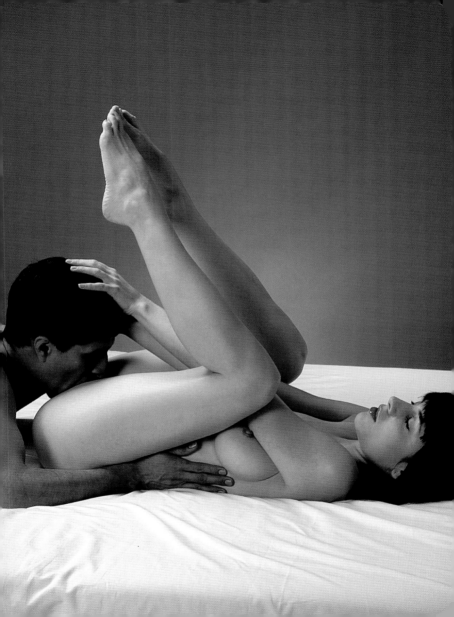

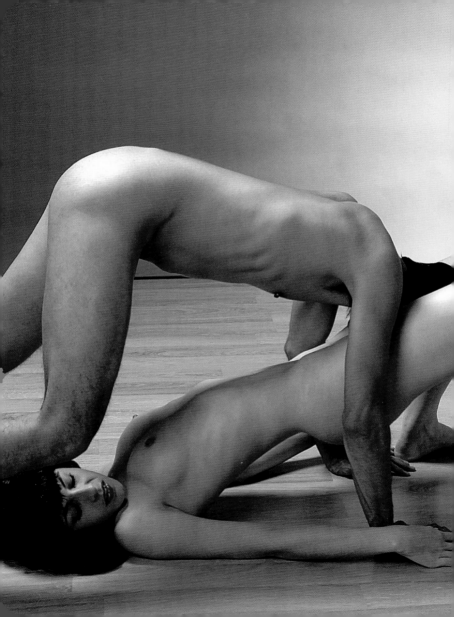

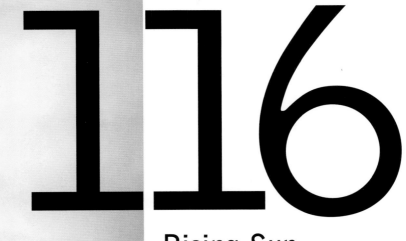

116

Rising Sun

Woman lies on her back with feet
on the floor lifting her hips to the ceiling.
Man goes on all fours, leaning his head
between her legs with his feet behind her
head. She undulates her pelvis,
rising up to meet him.

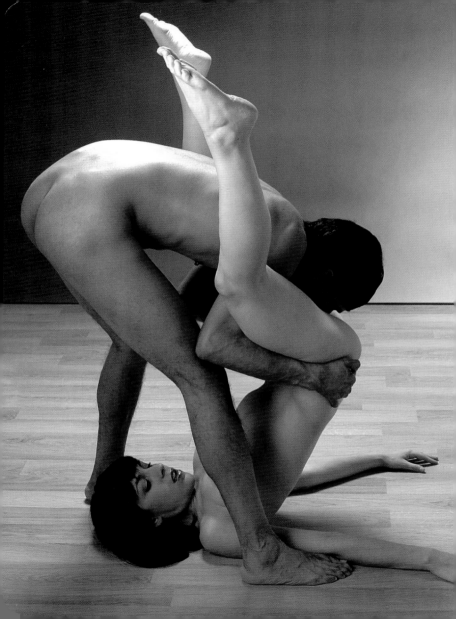

117

The Dip

With legs splayed, the man lifts the woman's
hips and legs in the air. Balancing against
each other, the man dips into her genitals
while he holds her firmly.

118

The Bird Feeder

Like The Dip, (117) the woman rests on her shoulders, her high legs in the air. This time he approaches facing her, his hands supporting her lower back, her legs on his shoulders. His face easily reaches her pleasure spots. She practices yoga while he practices his technique.

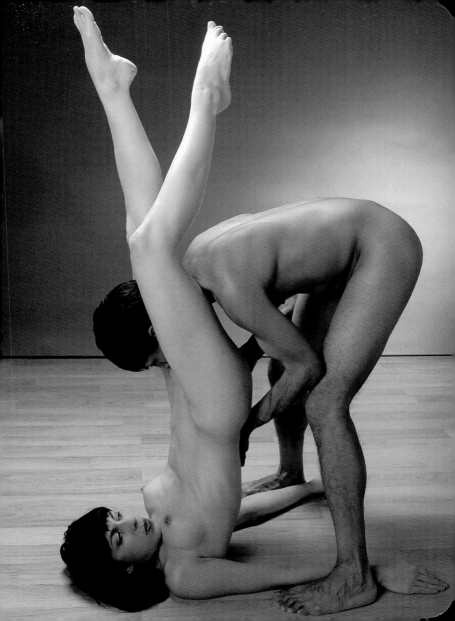

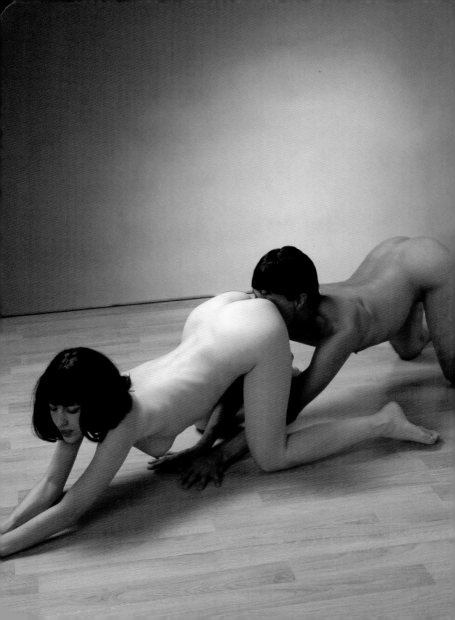

119

Chasing the Cat

The woman crawls on the floor, the man catches her on all fours, his face and arms in between her legs. For added spice, try this using a skateboard!

120

Seat of Honor

The man lies on his back. The woman takes her seat on his face, knees around his head, facing away from his body.

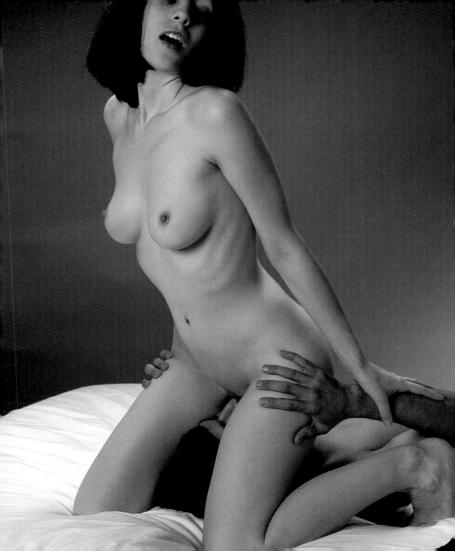

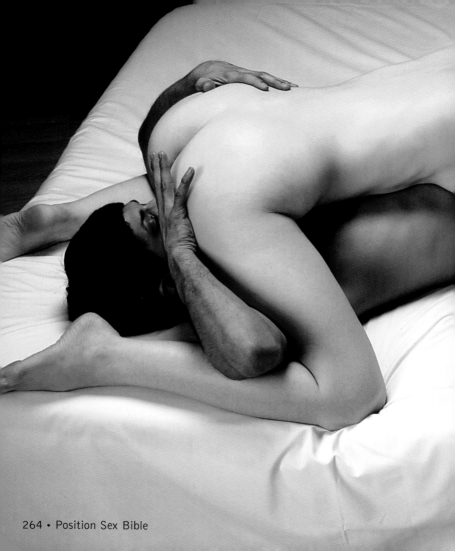

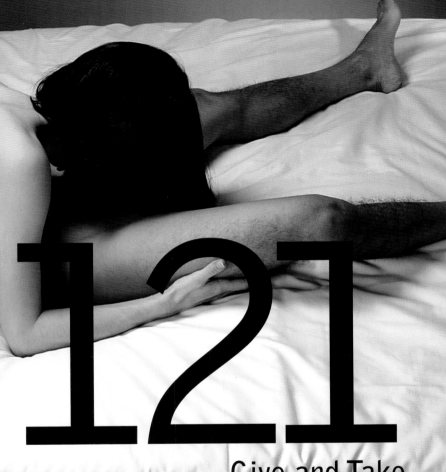

121

Give and Take

The man lies on his back. The woman lies over him with her vagina on his mouth. She takes his penis in her mouth. She undulates, controlling both ends of the situation.

122

Downtown Girl

(or Time-Tested)
The classic blow-job. The man stands with
the woman kneeling in front of him,
grasping his thighs.

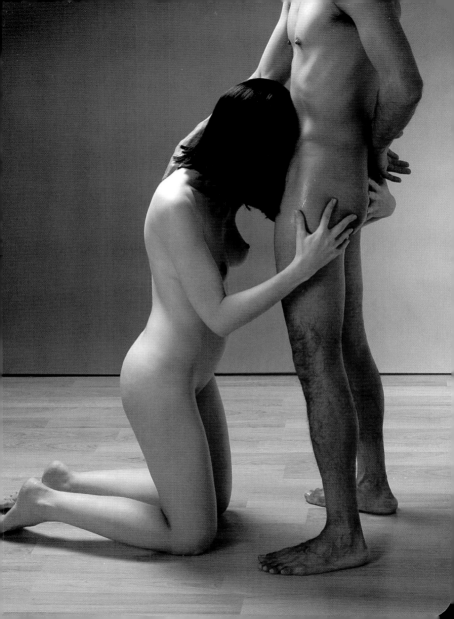

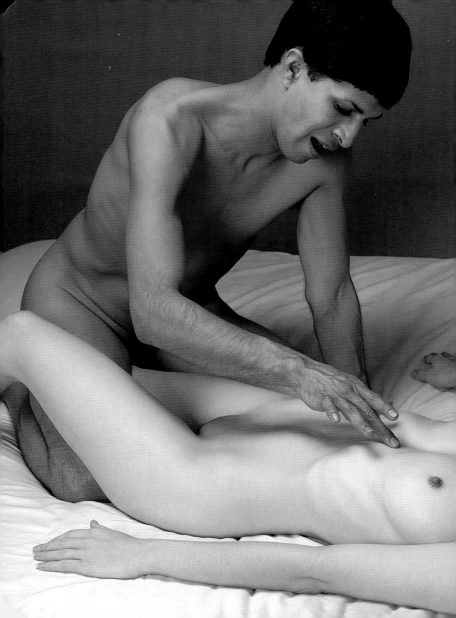

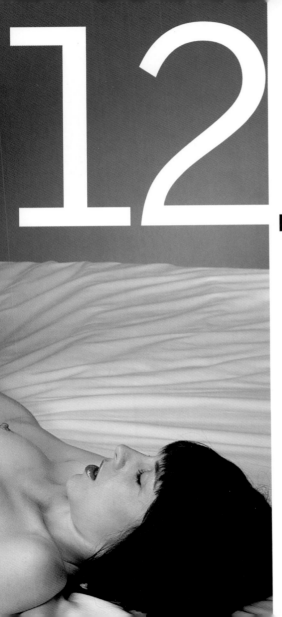

123

Slippery When Wet

With lubricated hands, the man kneels in front of the prone woman, massaging her torso with teasing light strokes. Will his hands move all the way down? He keeps her guessing.

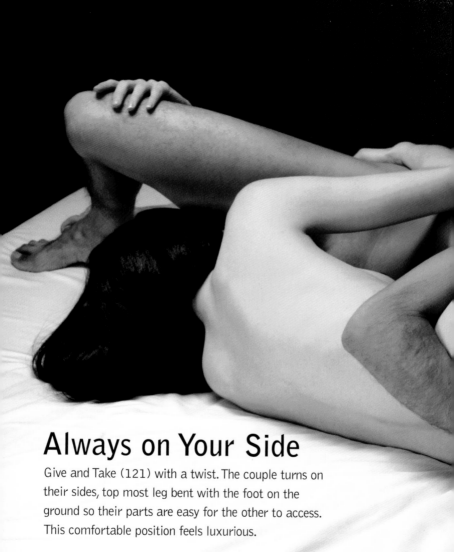

Always on Your Side

Give and Take (121) with a twist. The couple turns on their sides, top most leg bent with the foot on the ground so their parts are easy for the other to access. This comfortable position feels luxurious.

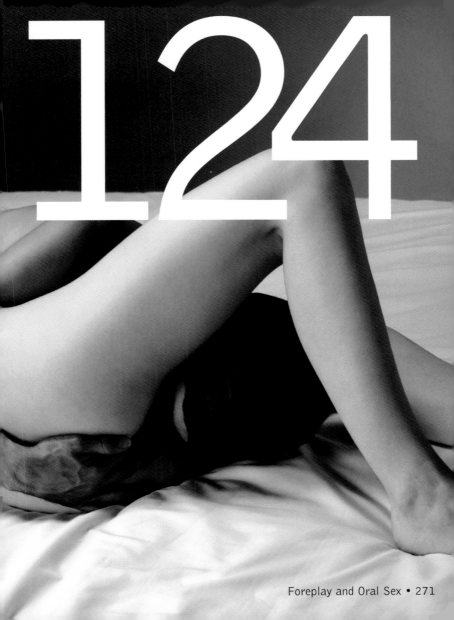

124

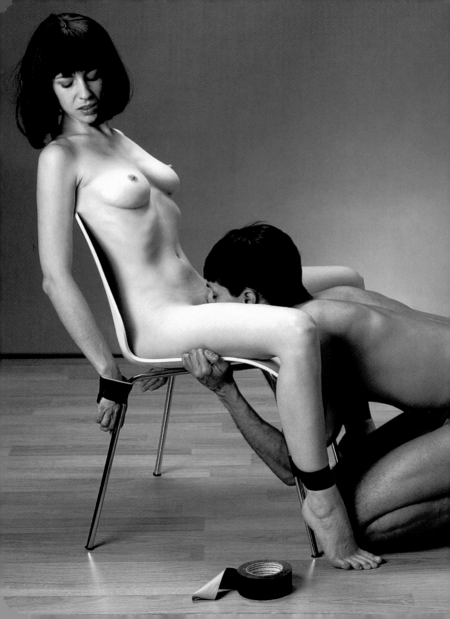

125

The Grateful Hostage

She sits in a chair, legs open, her ankles and wrists tied to the chair legs. He performs cunnilingus on his thankful prisoner.

126

A Bridge to Pleasure

The woman stands bending over so her hands are resting on the floor, her back arched like a cat. The man sits between her legs and stimulates her until he hears her mew.

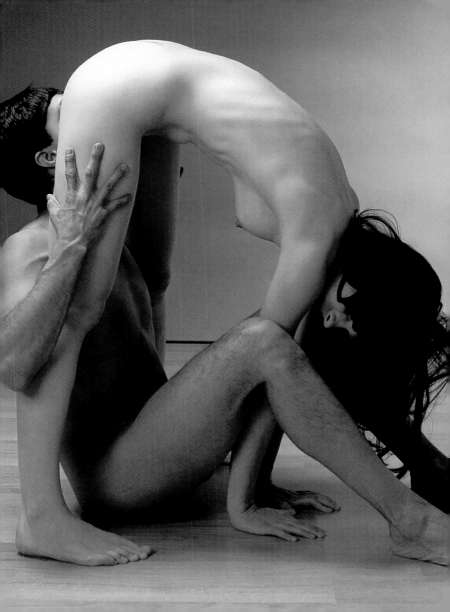

127

Tunnel of Love

She lies on her back. He squats over her placing
his penis between her lubricated breasts as she
holds them together creating a pleasing
"titty" tunnel of tightness.

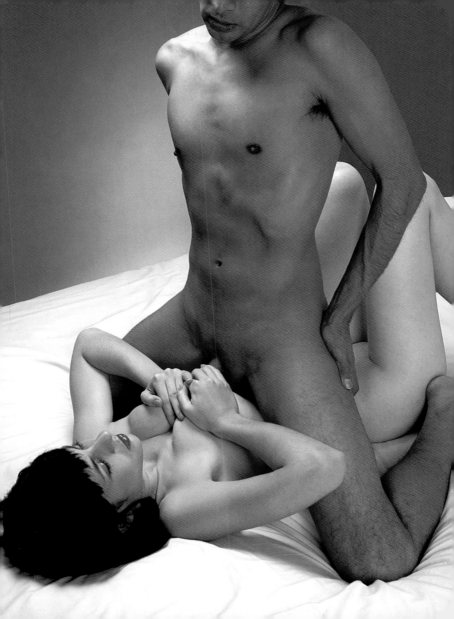

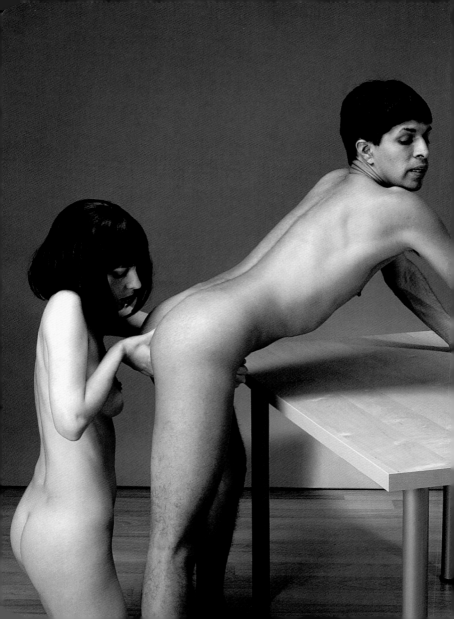

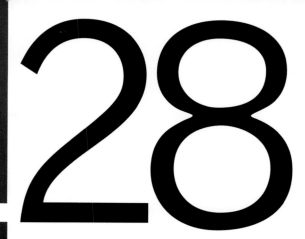

128

Checking the Oil

The man stands leaning on a table. The woman approaches him from behind, caressing his buttocks with her lubricated hands while she masturbates him.

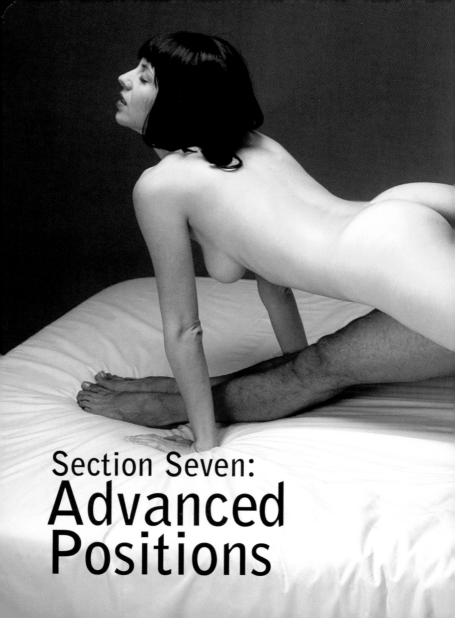

Section Seven:
Advanced
Positions

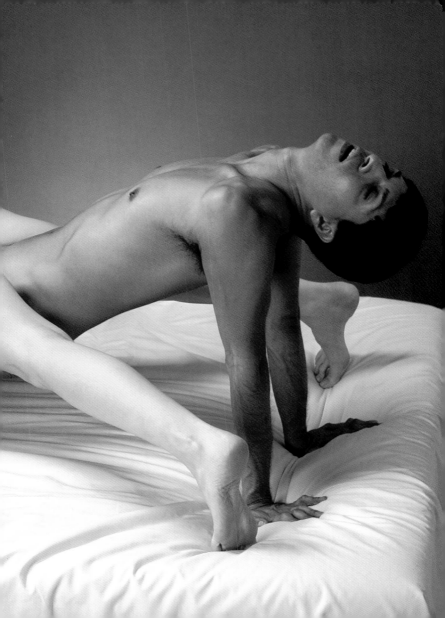

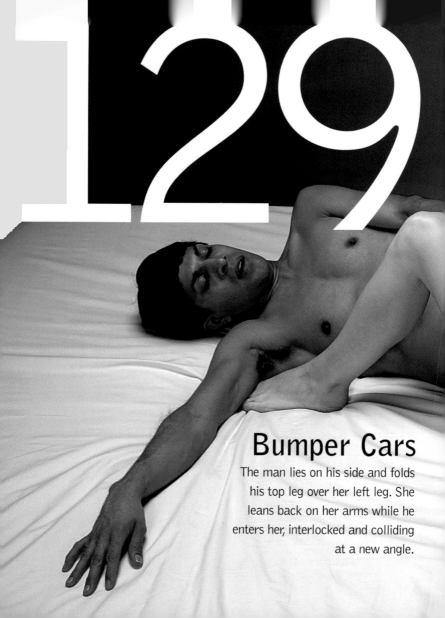

129

Bumper Cars

The man lies on his side and folds his top leg over her left leg. She leans back on her arms while he enters her, interlocked and colliding at a new angle.

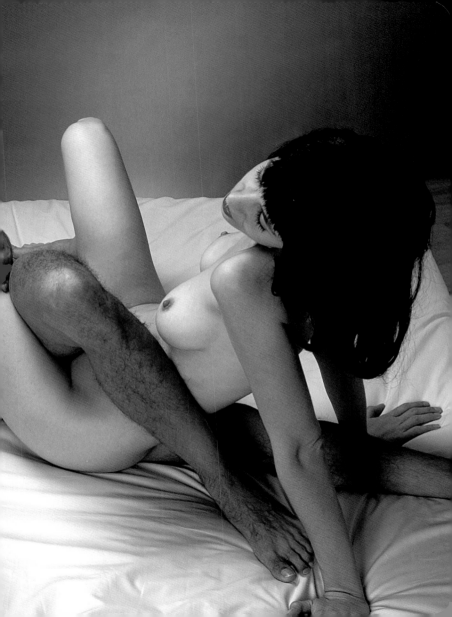

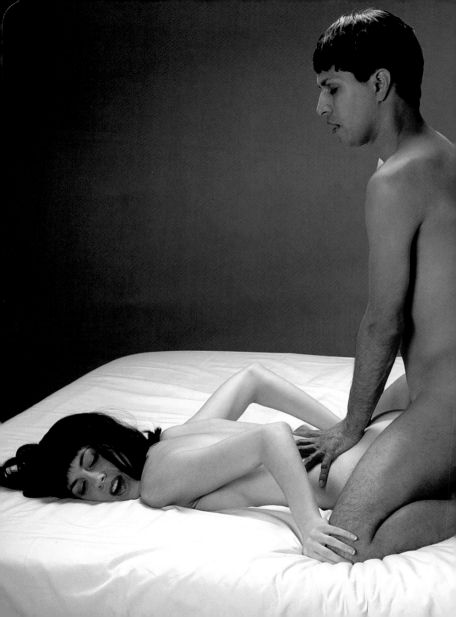

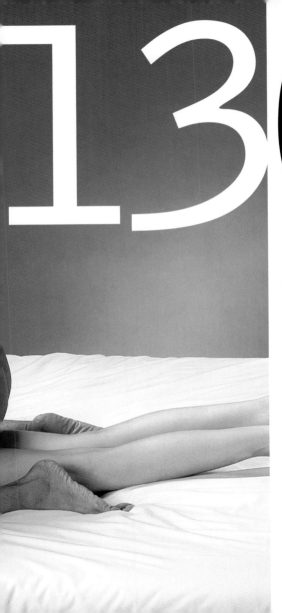

130

Back in the Saddle

The woman lies on her stomach. The man penetrates her from behind, deliciously stroking her back. She lifts up her buttocks to meet him.

131

The Plow

From The Tango (83), the woman wraps both legs around the man. She then arches backward and reaches and rests her hands on the floor. He continues thrusting until he plants his seed.

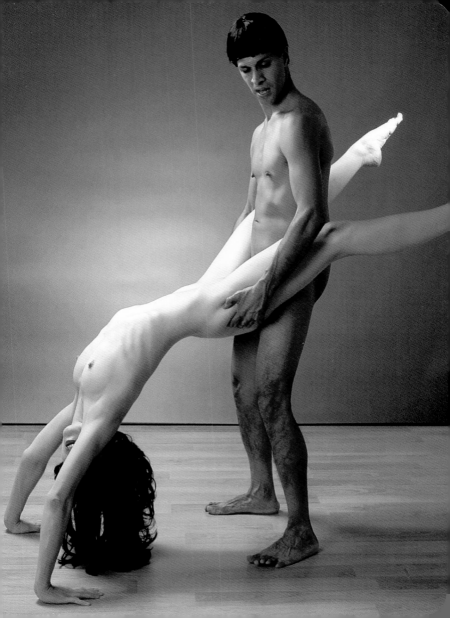

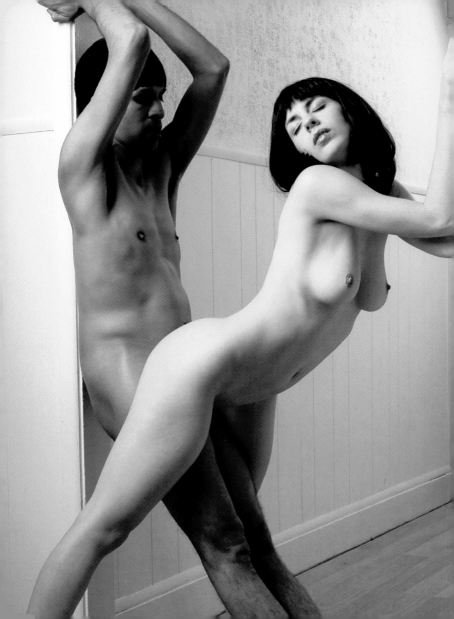

132

My Door Is Always Open

Man braces himself face up between a doorway, his back on one side and his feet on the opposite side. The woman straddles him leaning against the same side as his feet while he knocks pleasurably on her door.

133

The Nexus

The man kneels on the floor, sitting on his feet with his arms behind him on the floor for support. The woman approaches with the same leg position while he enters her. She leans back on her arms, allowing each of them to thrust back and forth.

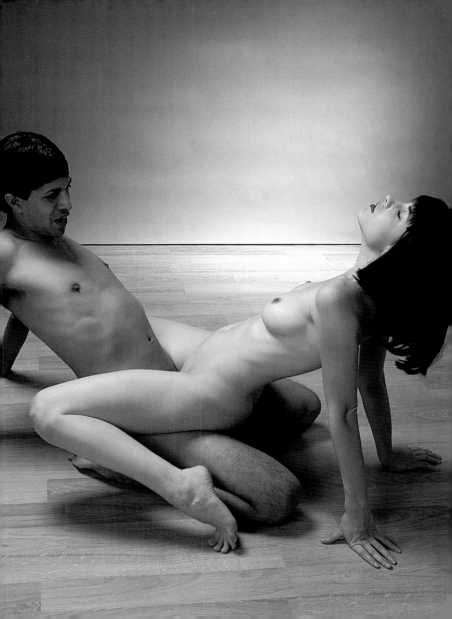

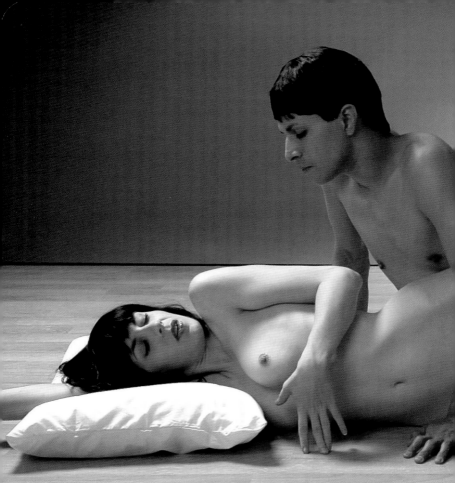

Elephants on Parade

While in the Baby Elephant (72), the woman
twists on her side, throwing her leg over the man.
He finds his way deep inside of her.

134

135

Table Saw

The woman holds herself horizontal, her right arm on floor, her right leg resting on a chair. Her left leg points to the ceiling while the man supports her back with his hands as he precisely guides himself to his mark.

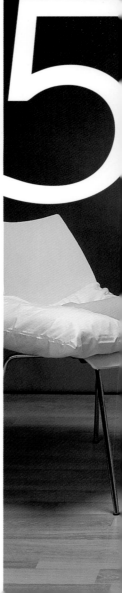

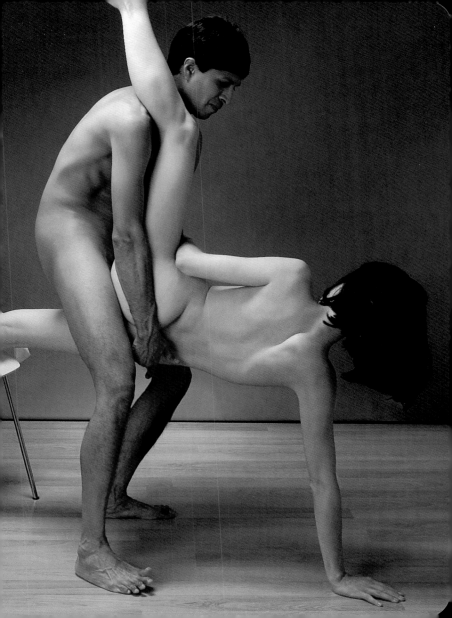

136

Queen of the World

While balanced in the Tug of War position (97),
the woman turns 180 degrees to face outward on
the man's lap. He holds her arms while she
stretches outward, calling forth favorable winds.

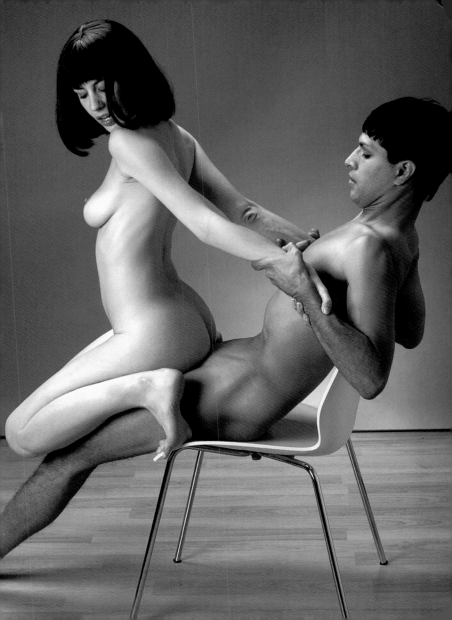

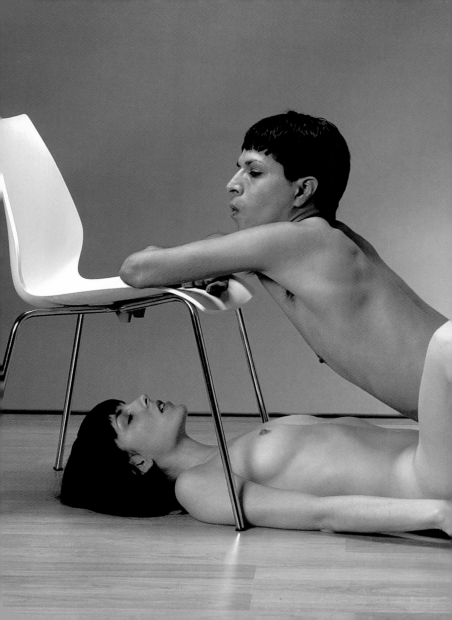

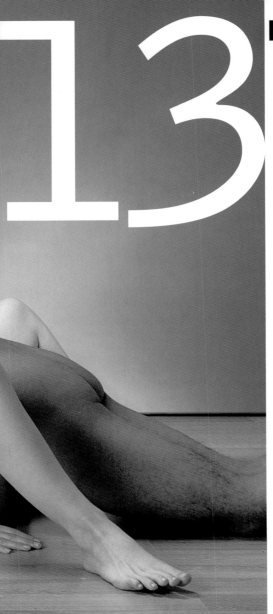

137

Fantasy City

In Straight-Edge Sex A (1) the addition of a chair acts as a barrier between the lovers. As the man rests his arms on the chair, he enters her at a 45-degree angle, giving them both a new perspective.

138

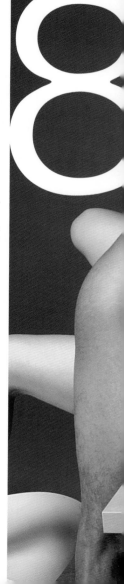

The Dinner Party

The woman lies on her back on a table, her leg resting on a chair or stool. The man stands at the edge of the table, straddling her leg and entering her as he leans over to sample her treats.

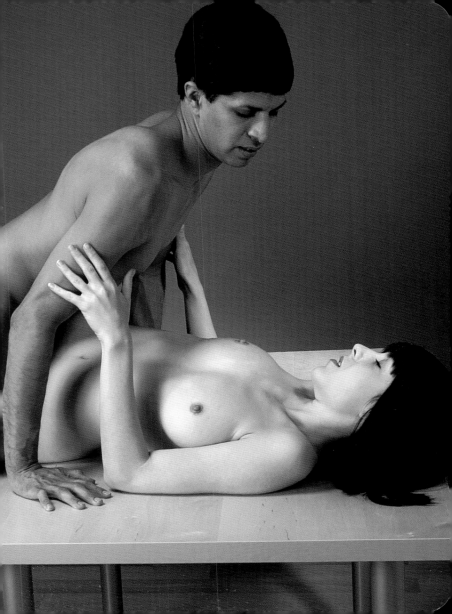

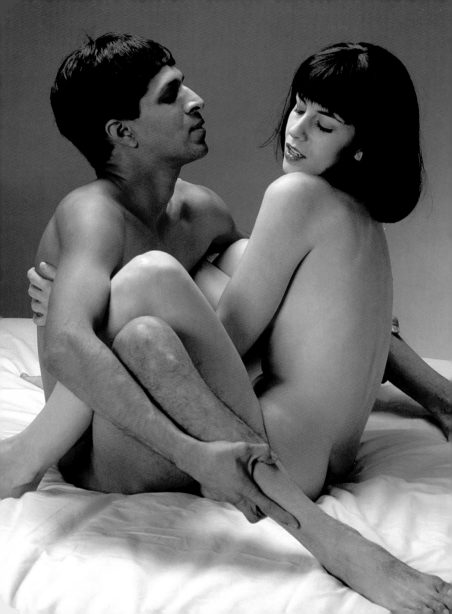

139

The Kissing Lotus

Moving from The Crab (17), the man intertwines his legs with hers. They are now kissing distance while they make love.

140

The Sheath

A reclining variation on the standing
Hoover (87). The man seats himself while
inside his lover. She drapes herself over his
lap and pushes up against the floor. Not
for the weak of tricep.

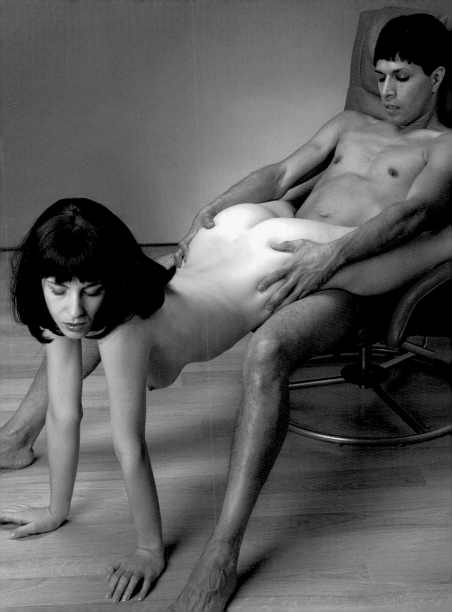

141

Members Only Entrance

The man leans against a doorpost and invites the woman to climb aboard. She straddles him holding on to his neck, and he braces himself for the ride.

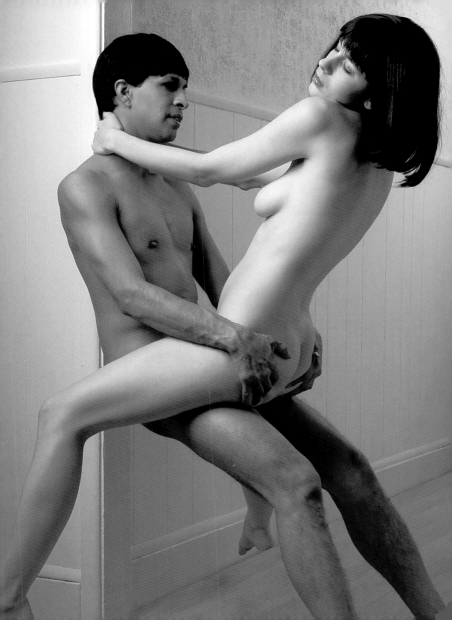

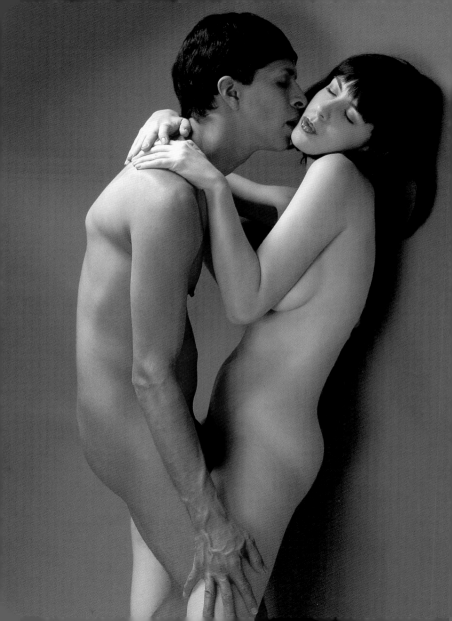

142

Lean on Me

The woman leans back against the wall. The man faces the woman standing in between her legs. The woman captures her lover's weight while he dips and raises himself in and out of her.

143

The Consolation

The classic doggy-style with equipment.
The woman lies face down on a chair and
the man enters her from behind. Great for
G-spot stimulation. Don't forget the pillow
for the knees!

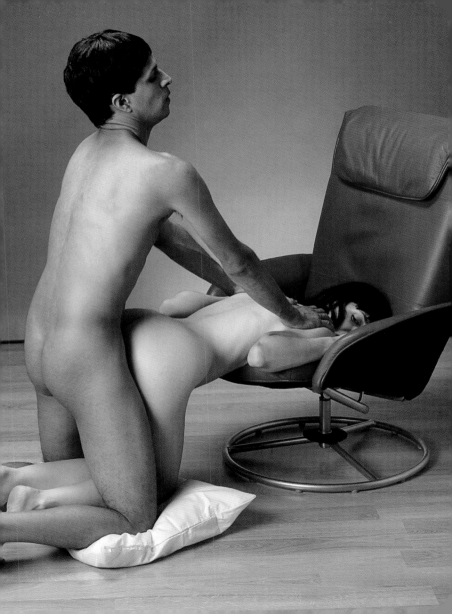

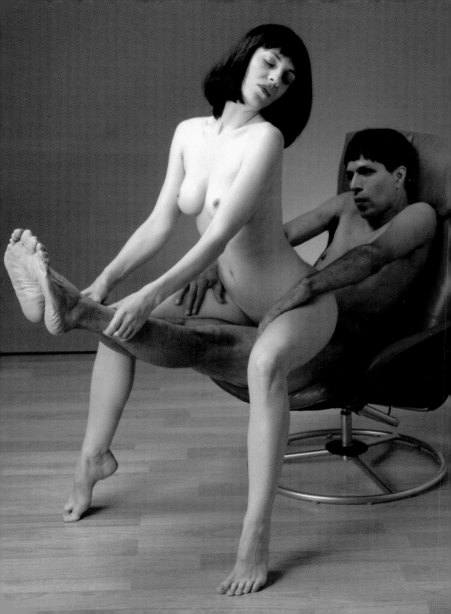

144

The Lady Godiva

Using a rocking chair or the edge of the
bed, the woman sits on her lover's lap
facing away from him and pulls his legs
up between hers. They let the motion of
the chair rock them to climax.

145

The Bare Hug

Like the Sitting Body Wrap (75), the woman sits on the
man's lap pressing her body against his.
This position allows her to control the movement by
pushing her feet downward on the chair.

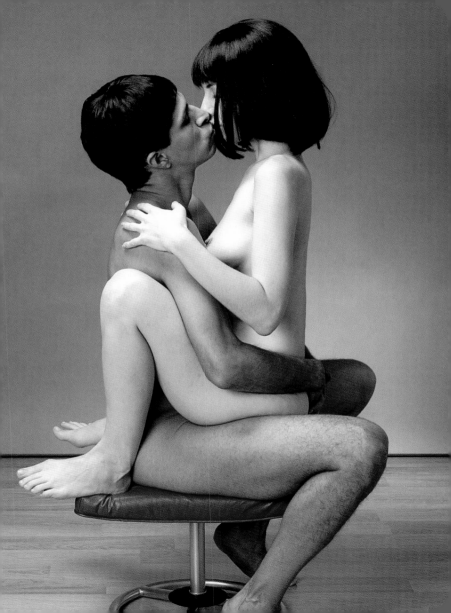

146

Cupid's Bow

Starting from Come Sit on My Lap (98), the man stands supporting the woman at a right angle at hip level. Her legs are folded against him. He grasps her hands tightly to keep her safe. Only for the agile in mind and body.

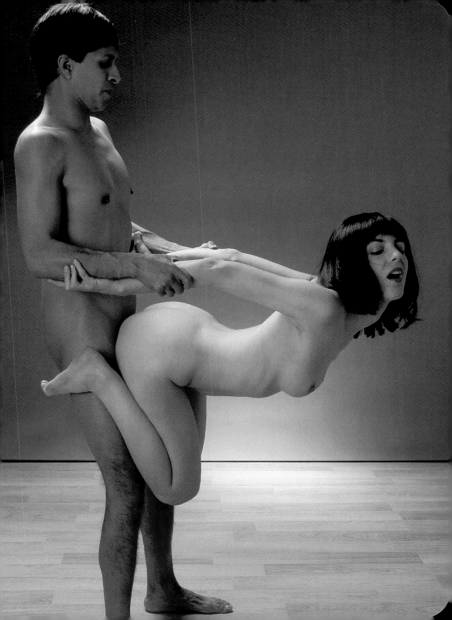

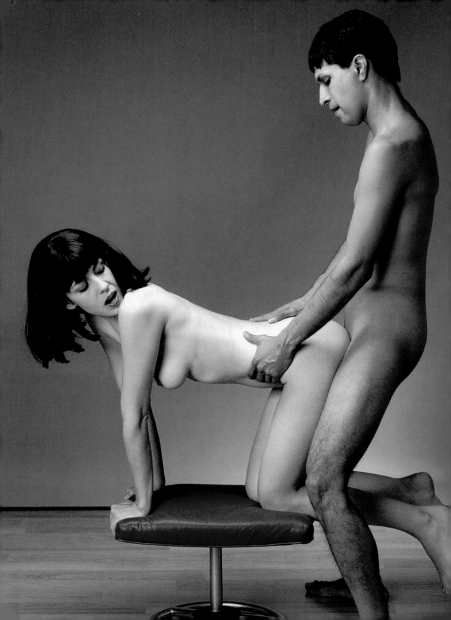

147

Tight Quarters

The woman kneels across an armless chair, her hands on one side, her knees on the other. The man penetrates deeply from behind.

148

I've Found My Niche

The woman leans face-first into a door jam. The man
leans back against the opposite side, his feet braced
where she's leaning. He straddles her right leg. Her
left leg is bent and rests on his left leg.

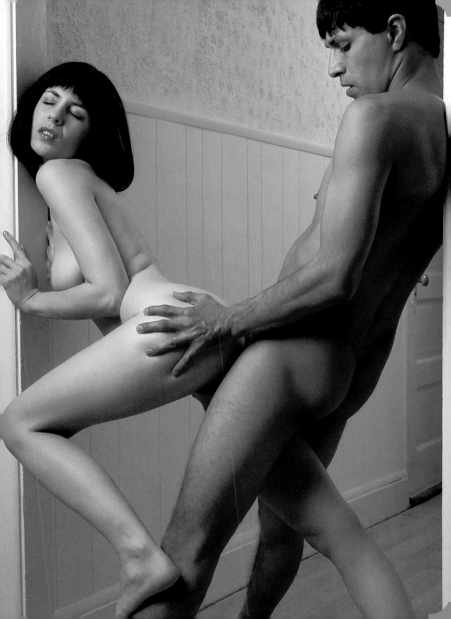

149

The Long and Deep of It

The woman lies facedown on a rocking chair with knees on the floor. The man enters her from behind as he holds one leg up. Deep penetration for him, increased clitoral stimulation for her.

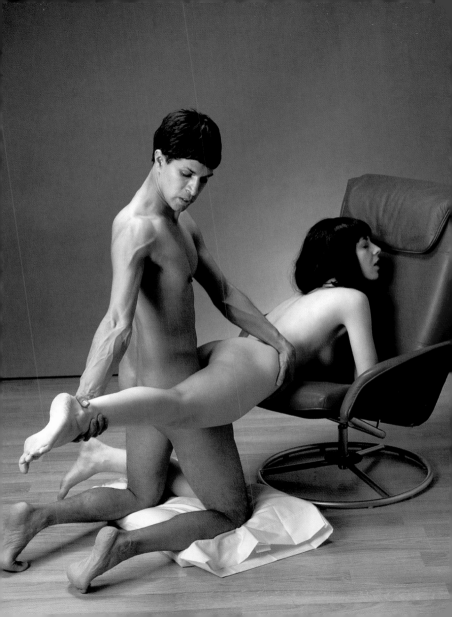

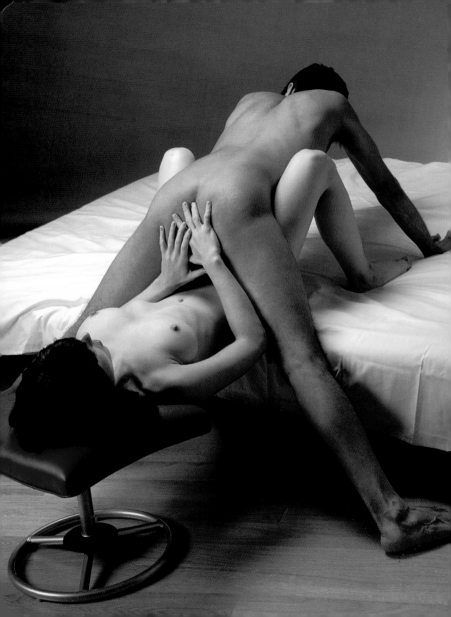

150

Into Each, His Own

The couple is interlocked with the woman lying across a footstool and a bed. With her arms free, the woman can fondle the man's testicles as she stimulates her clitoris as well.

151

The Door Jam

Propped against the door jam like My Door Is Always Open (132), this time the woman faces her lover, allowing them to kiss as she presses into him. His solid stance gives her freedom of movement.

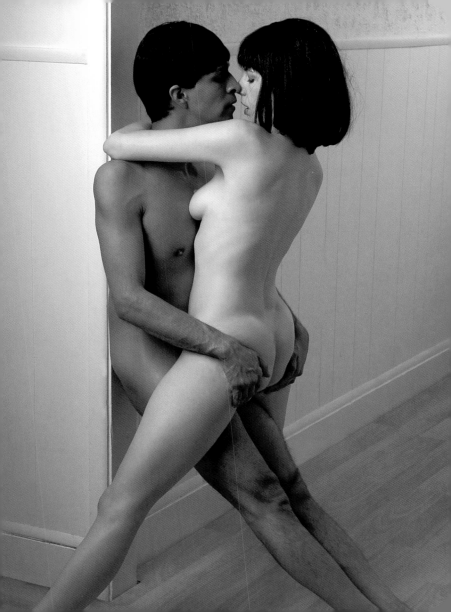

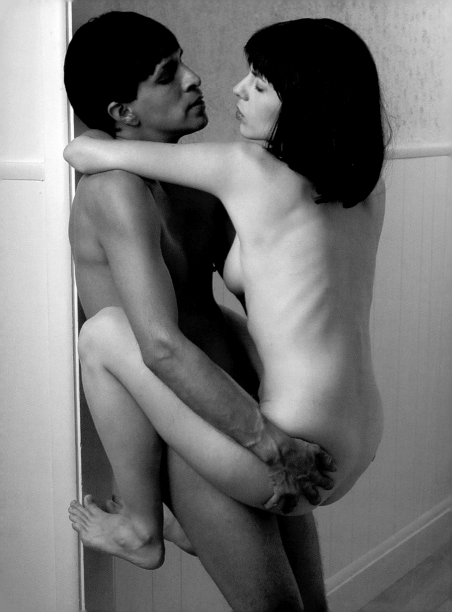

152

Climbing the Walls

From The Door Jam (151) she climbs
aboard, her feet against the wall as he
supports her weight. He can move deeply
inside her as she clings to him.

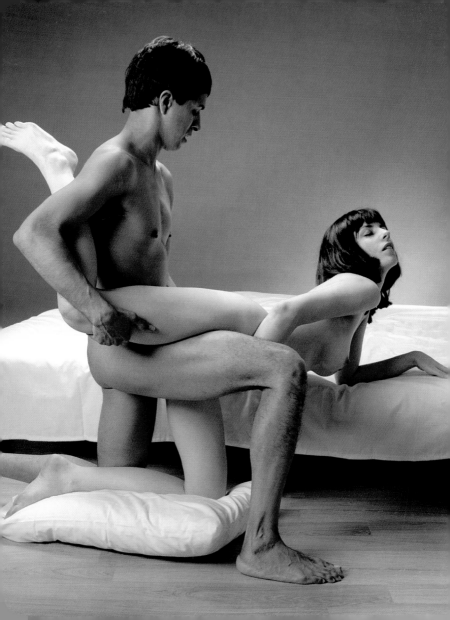

153

Synchronized Deep Diving

From The Long and Deep of It (149), he raises her leg higher, supporting it on his bent right knee. The bed acts as a buffer and he can thrust even deeper into her.

154

Long Night, Full Moon

Woman leans in a rocking chair, her butt on
the edge of the chair, her feet on the floor.
He lies across her body, supporting himself on
his elbows. Her free hands can caress his legs,
buttocks, and testicles.

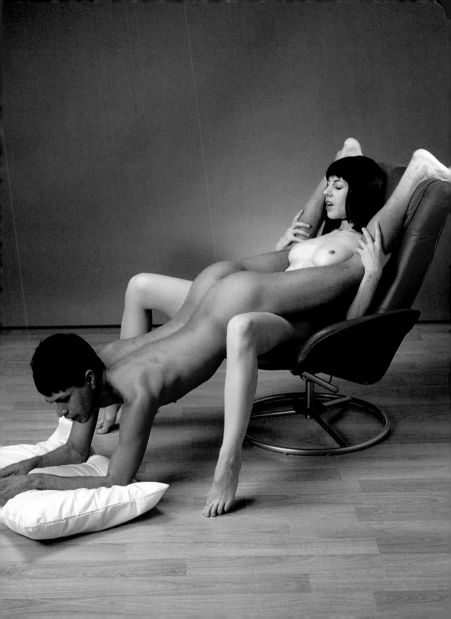

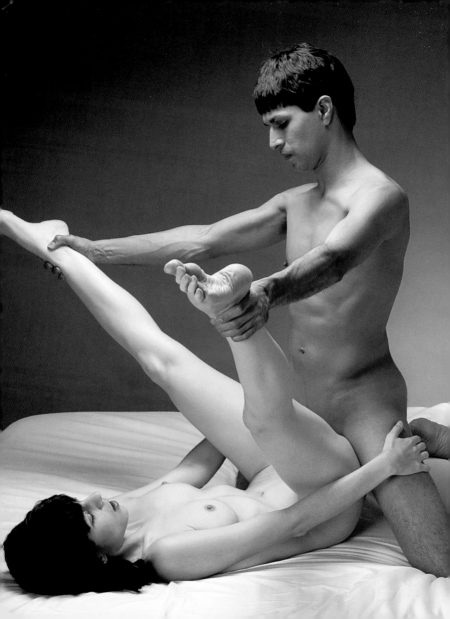

155

Spreading Some Joy

She is on her back. He kneels and enters her, holding a firm group on her ankles. Her legs are wide open, giving him a clear view of her genitals as he watches himself move in and out.

156

Deep Satisfaction

The woman does a modified headstand, careful
to support her neck and head with her hands.
She leans over to give her man full access to her
as he holds her steady and enters her from
behind. She can't see what he'll do, leaving her
with just the sensation of his thrusting.

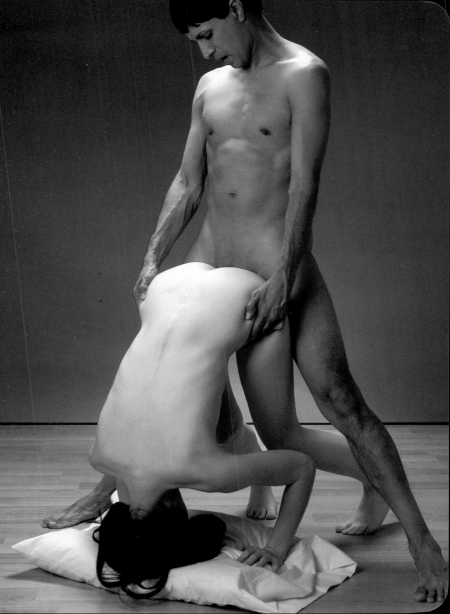

157

Surfing the Wave

The man lies down faceup. His lover lowers herself sideways on him. Both have a hand free and easy access to rubbing her clitoris.

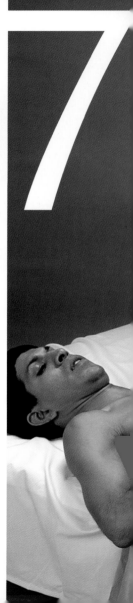

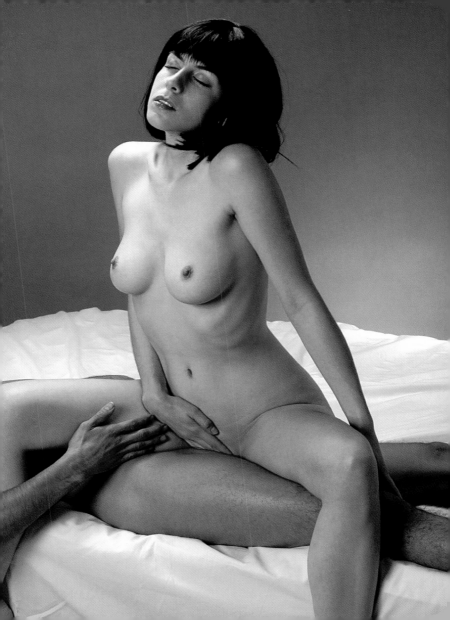

158

Leapfrog

A simple hop into her lover's lap offers
the woman an opportunity for G-spot
activation. She controls the movements
while he massages her back.

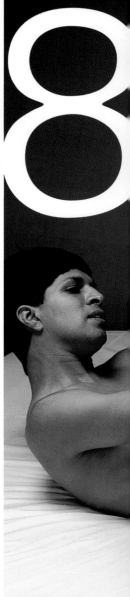

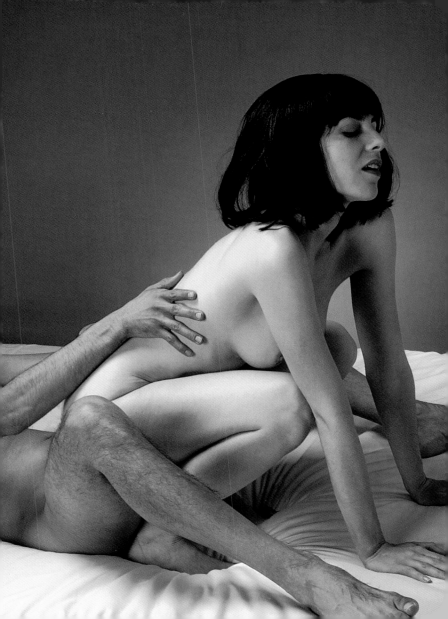

159

Blooming Lotus

From The Kissing Lotus (139), the couple spread their bodies apart, leaning back on their hands. This position allows the point of penetration to be lower down, conferring new sensations with each movement.

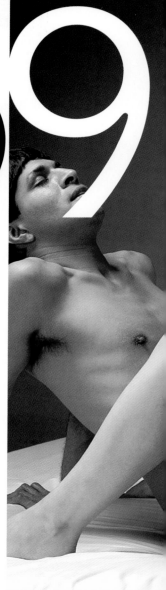

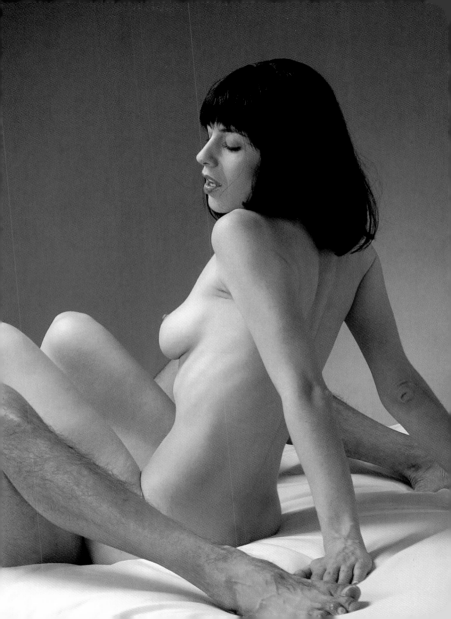

160

Speaking in Tongues

He lies on his back on the bed. The woman squats over her lover's face, resting on his knees with her hands. He kisses her genitals while she moves back and forth, helping her to orgasm.

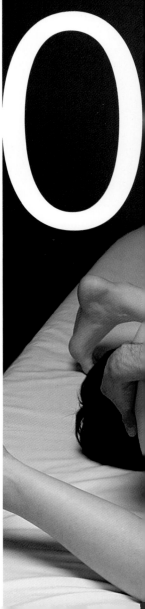

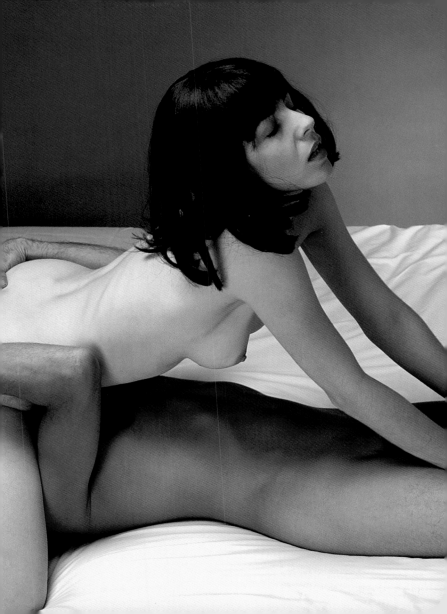

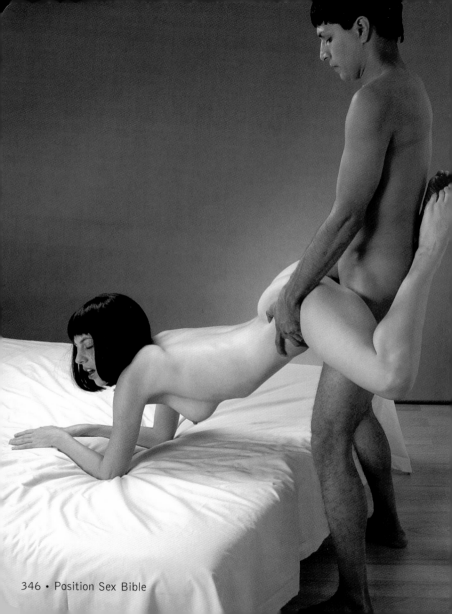

161

The Nail-Gun

He stands on the floor facing the bed, knees
slightly bent. She leans on the bed as he
holds her by the hips, her legs straddling him.
Her knees are bent behind him, her heels on
his upper back. He finds his target each time.

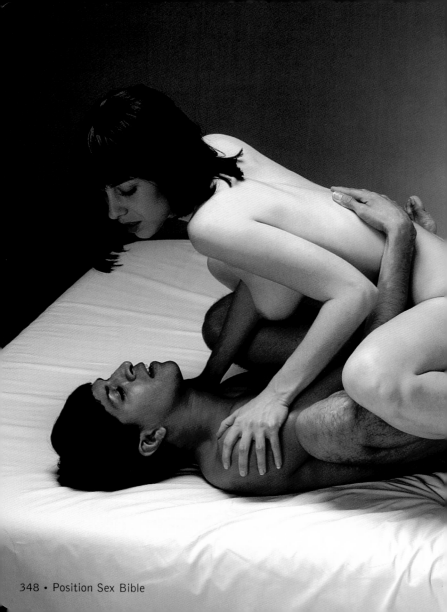

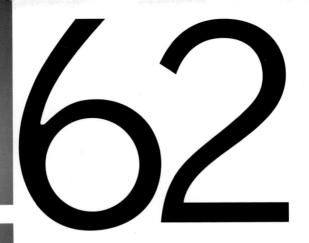

162

Praying Mantis

The man is on his back on the bed with his legs up and knees bent. The woman crouches on top of him. She squats to meet his penis as it disappears inside of her.

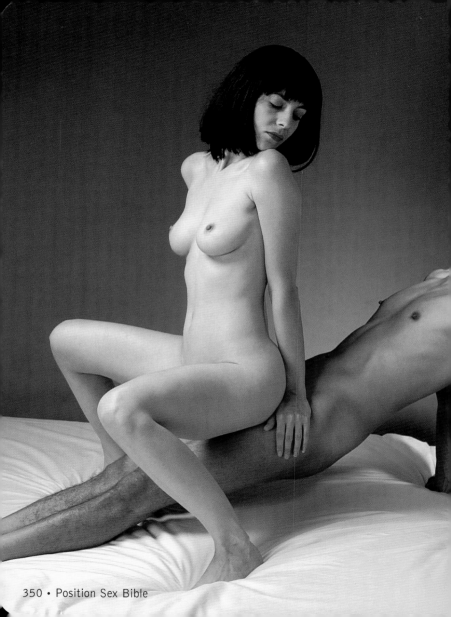

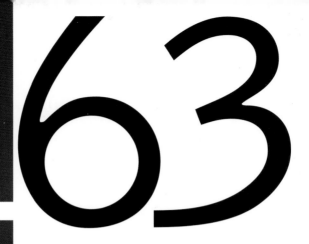

163

Lowered Inhibition

The man assumes the yoga bridge position. The woman lowers herself onto him, leaning against his hips. She can bounce up and down using her legs as leverage.

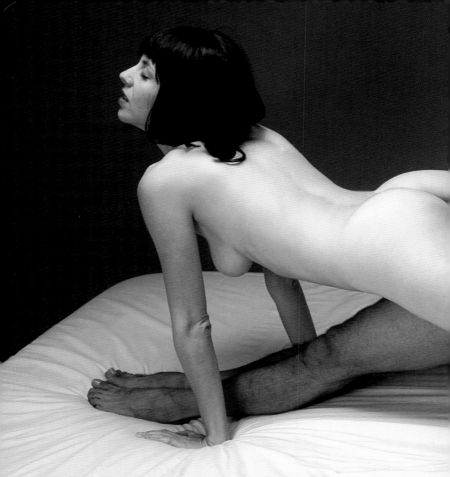

Meet Me in the Middle

Moving from Lowered Inhibition (163), the woman faces the opposite direction from the man and assumes a modified yoga cobra position. They are joined only in the middle, creating a large X with their bodies.

164

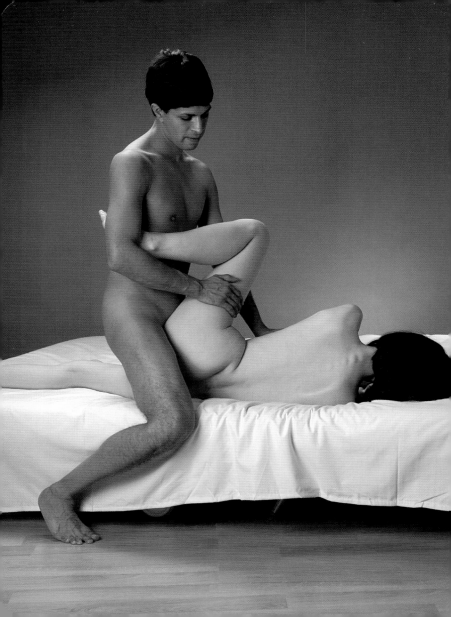

165

Studying Geometry

She lies on the bed near the edge on her side with one leg on the floor. He straddles her bottom leg, holding her top leg up and against his body. He pushes into her at a whole new angle.

166

Behind the Scenes

The man enters from the rear as she kneels on a footstool, leaning against a table or chair. He uses one hand to caress her buttocks as his other moves her back and forth.

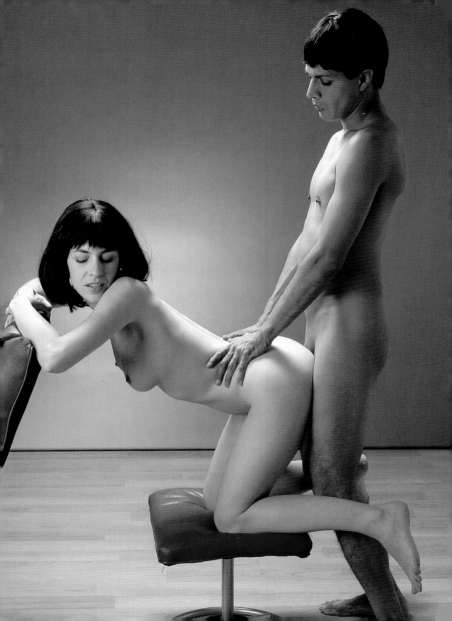

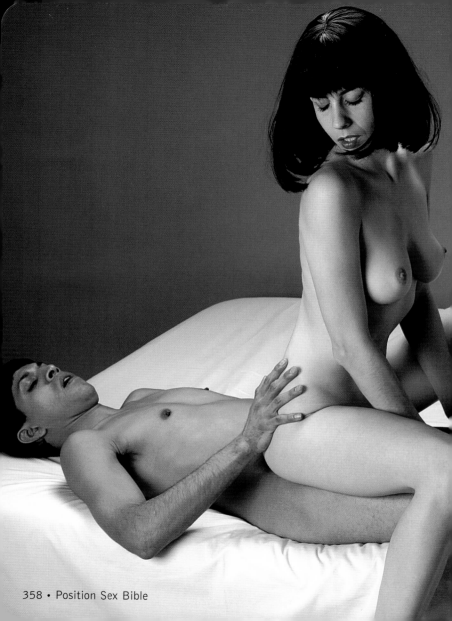

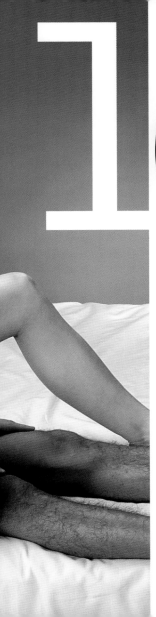

167

Hopping the Fence

The man is at the edge of the bed so his lover can hop aboard. With her legs spread, she has access to both her own parts and his.

168

I Saved Your Seat

Difficult but worthwhile, the woman leans back and provides a place for her lover to "sit." He enters her while supporting himself with his arms on the floor. An unforgettable position.

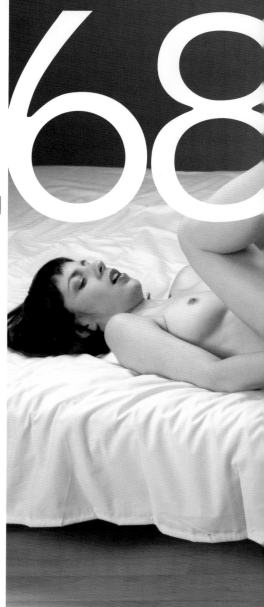

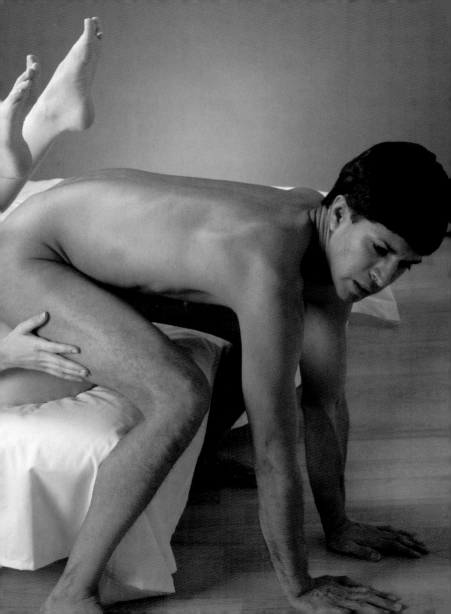

169

Upside Down You Turn Me

She lies on the bed on her back, her legs together and raised toward the ceiling. He faces the opposite direction, backing into her, his legs straddling her body. She pulls him in closer and he rocks back and forth on his elbows.

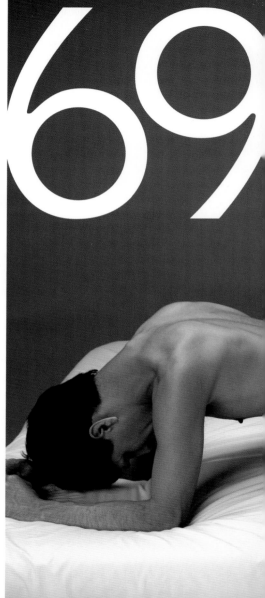

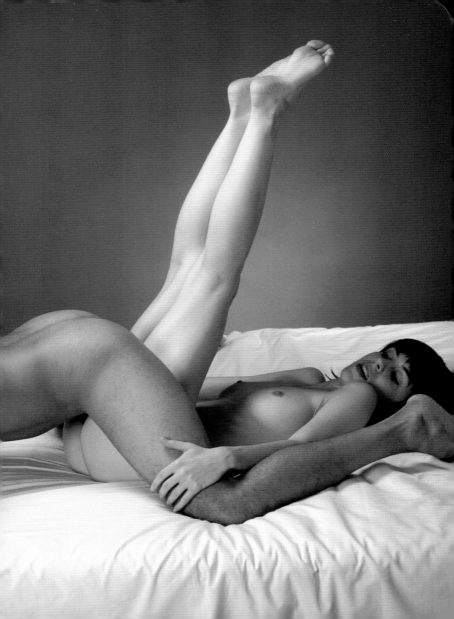

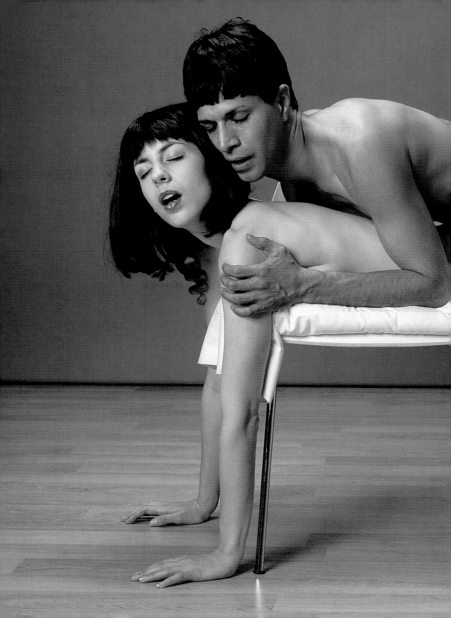

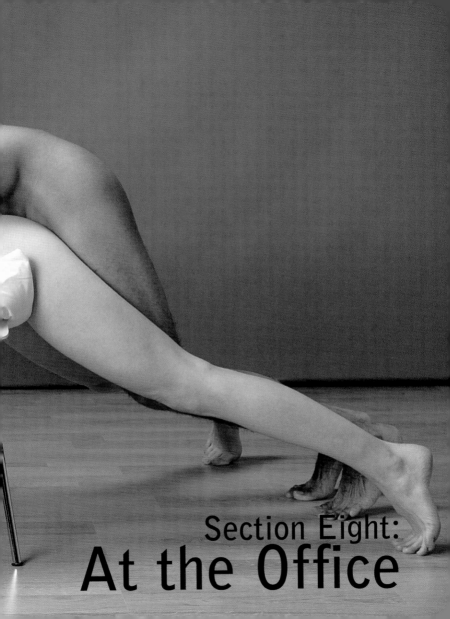

Section Eight:
At the Office

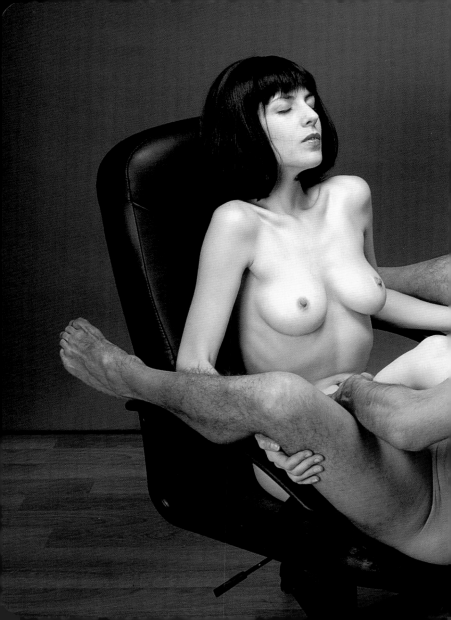

170

The Corporate Merger

She's in the seat of power, asking him to join her company. He leans back against the desk, their bodies merged as one. His hands are free to provide extra service.

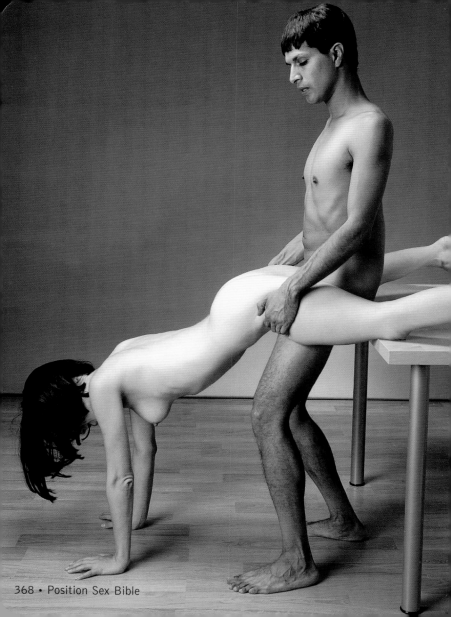

171

The Motivator

The Hoover (87) with a little office support. His buttocks and her legs are supported by the table. He gives a taste of her year-end bonus.

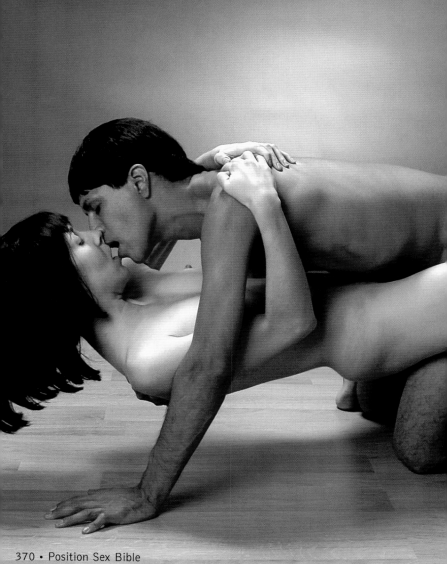

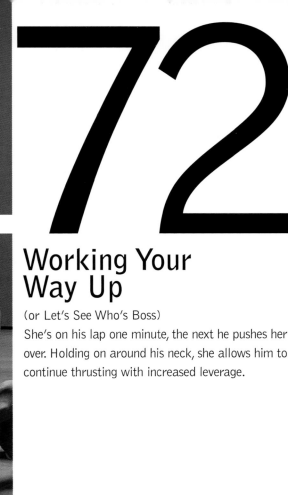

172

Working Your Way Up

(or Let's See Who's Boss)

She's on his lap one minute, the next he pushes her over. Holding on around his neck, she allows him to continue thrusting with increased leverage.

173

Out of the Box

The woman goes into a modified yoga shoulder stand, while the man takes advantage of her openness. He gently offers a new way of looking at things.

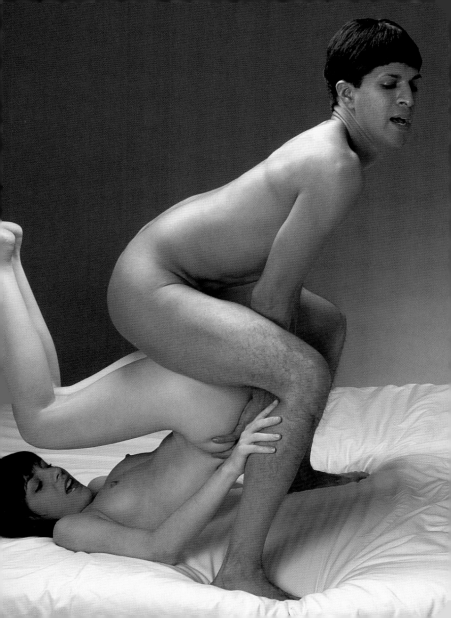

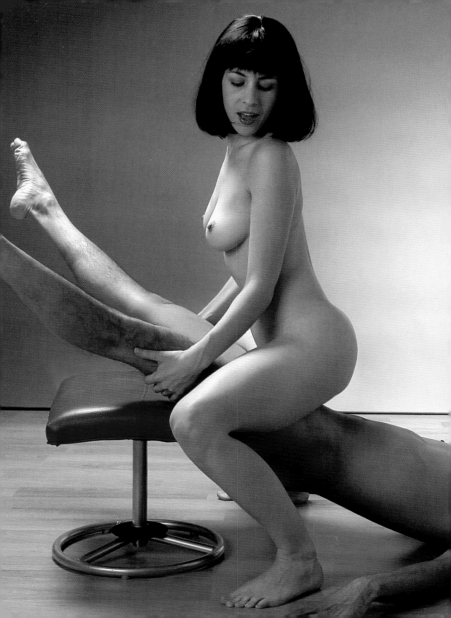

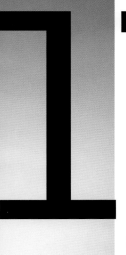

174

Power Broker

She sends the profit line straight up as she straddles her lover. He supports himself while he lets her ride the momentum.

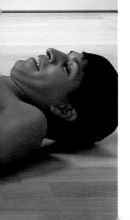

175

Giving Her a Raise

After he claims her on the bed, the woman is raised up and fully supported. Her feet are wrapped around her lover's head. They use their arms to come closer.

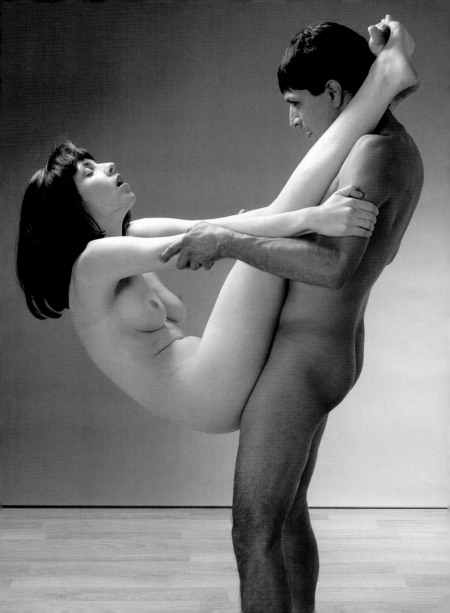

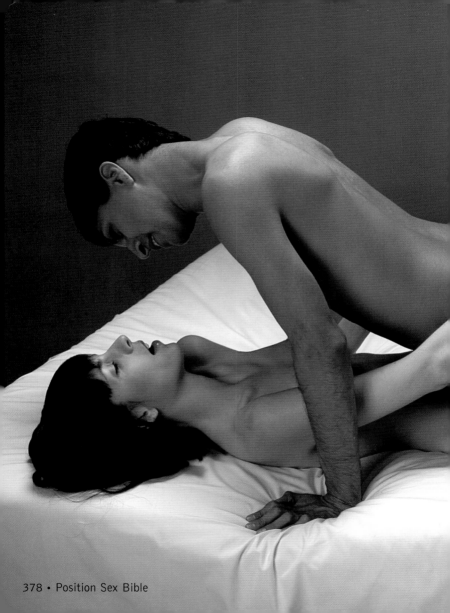

176

Entry-Level Position

While engaging in sex in the classic missionary position, the woman stimulates the man's hind parts. This double-entry position provides bonus pleasure for both lovers.

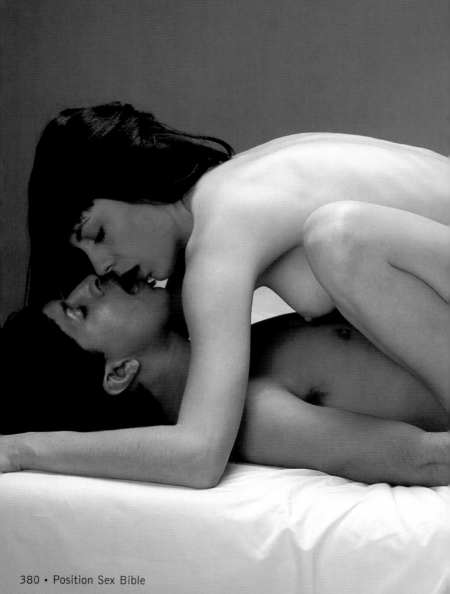

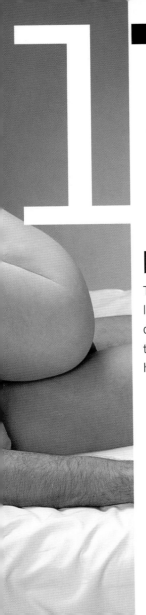

177

Loving Takeover

The woman takes charge, crouching over her lover's body. In this position, the vagina is fully open, allowing for deeper penetration. She can take over her own pleasuring by rubbing herself against her lover as she moves.

178

Climbing the Ladder

Climbing on a chair, and each other, the couple
engage in rear penetration. Be careful not to tip
over as you make your way to the top.

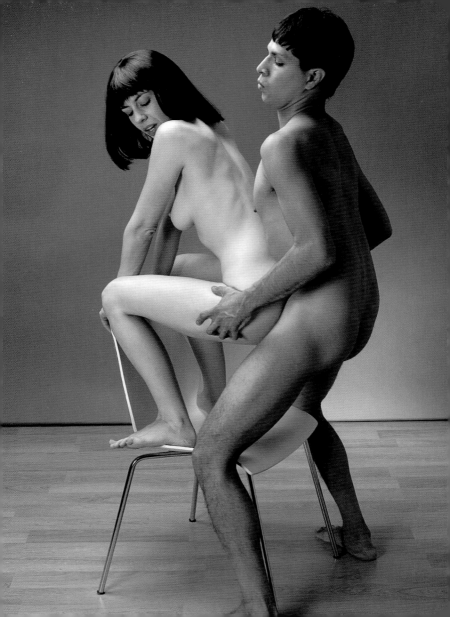

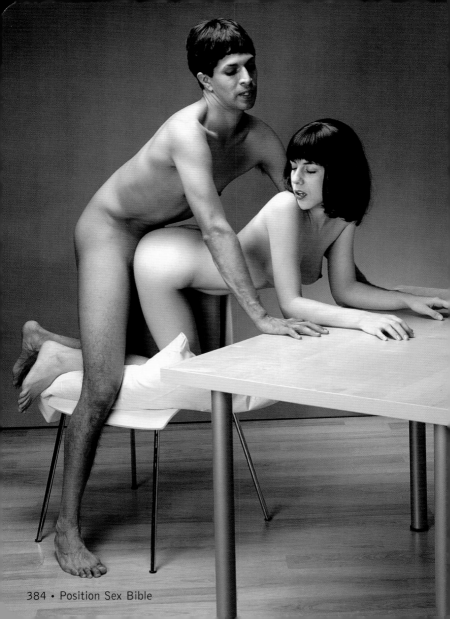

179

Behind on Work

Using a desk and chair, the woman leans forward onto the desk. The man straddles the chair, and gets to work from behind. Recommended for after-hours catch-up only.

180

Flex Benefits

Because the woman is bridging between the chair and the bed, she is free to be flexible with how her lover enters her. He can drape one leg over her and twist himself to make it work.

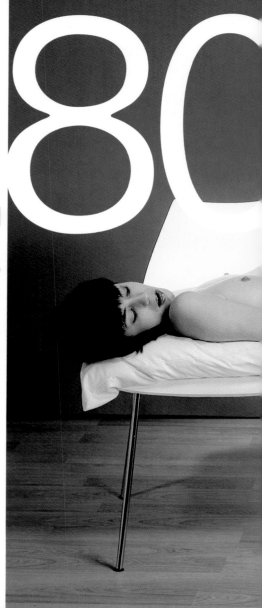

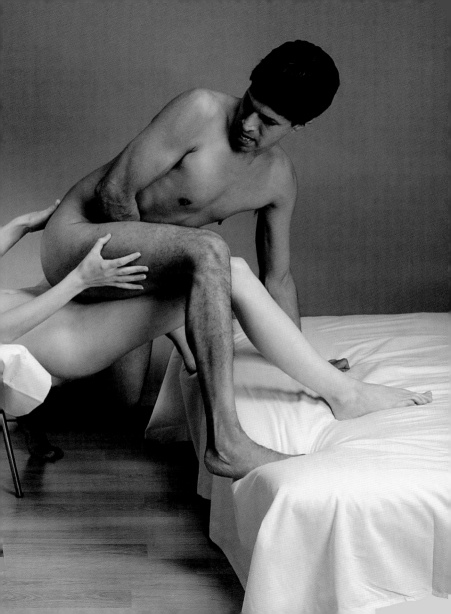

181

Double Shift

He enters her from behind while leaning back
against a wall. She brings his hands around to
her clitoris, instructing him in the best way to
pleasure her. They can time their orgasms to
clock out at the end of their shift.

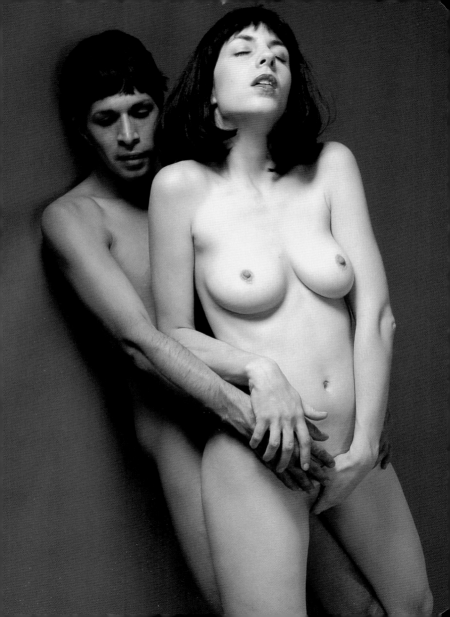

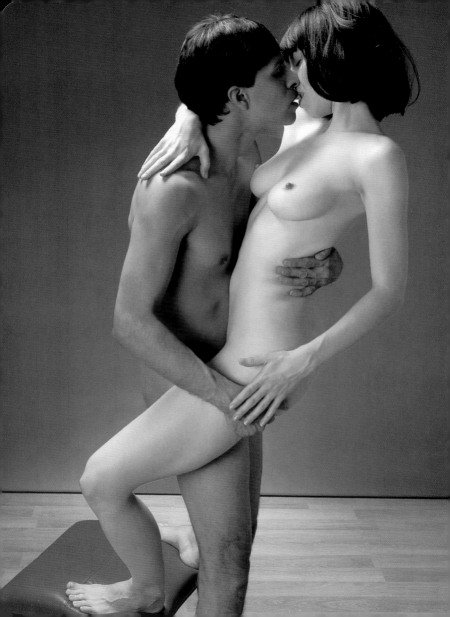

182

The Profit Share

The woman is supported by her lover, while she wraps herself around him. She uses a footstool to rest her feet, relieving the man of some of his supporting duties. The footstool helps the lovers merge.

Take a
Letter Please

The man is on the edge of his chair, leaning
back, feet braced against the desk. The woman
backs into him while pushing against the desk.

183

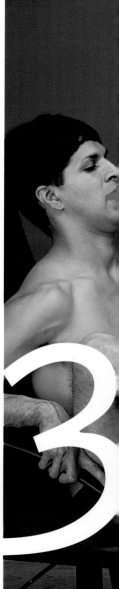

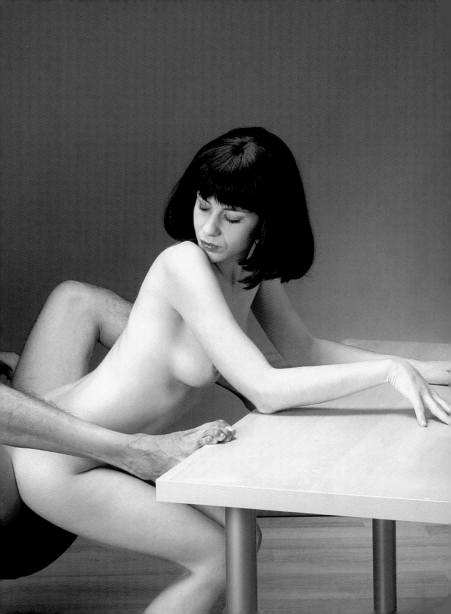

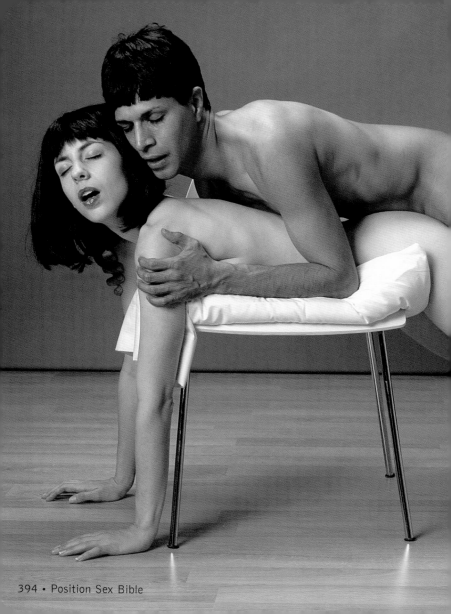

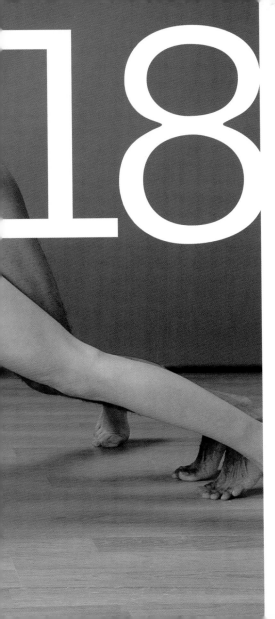

184

Sharing Your Assets

Another opportunity for a complete merger. The chair lifts her off the ground to meet her lover's body as they share their pleasure.

185

Squeeze Me In

The woman curls up in a ball on the desk,
facedown. The man casually walks up and
lets himself in.

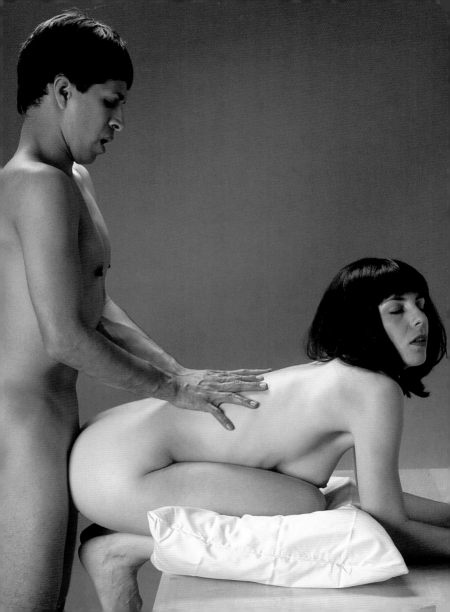

186

The Ruthless Negotiator

The woman lies back on a footstool, legs in the air. She leaves the man no choice but to make a counteroffer.

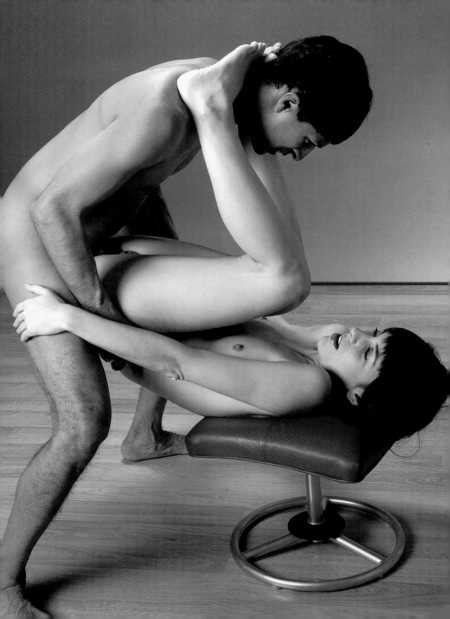

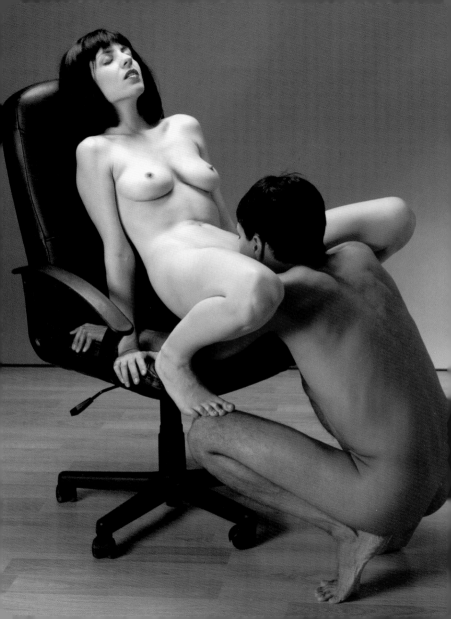

187

Appealing to Your Target Market

Right on target, the couple converge. With the woman crouching, she can press against her lover bringing his mouth to her. They have one goal in mind.

188

Better Than Phone Sex

She sits on the edge of the desk leaning back on her arms. He stands before her and enters her while caressing her breasts.

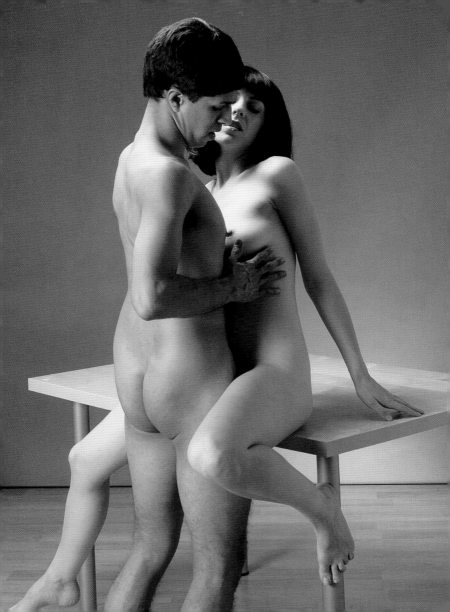

189

Tight Schedule

Even with a heavy deadline, there's time
for a quickie. She leans forward on the
desk, her buttocks thrust out, one leg
raised, giving him easy access to the
break in her schedule.

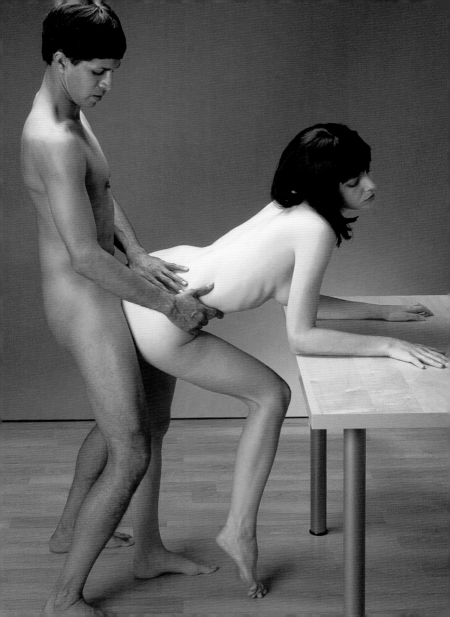

190

Getting the Memo

Classic, but still exciting. He's in his chair. She's under the desk, bringing the project to its climactic conclusion.

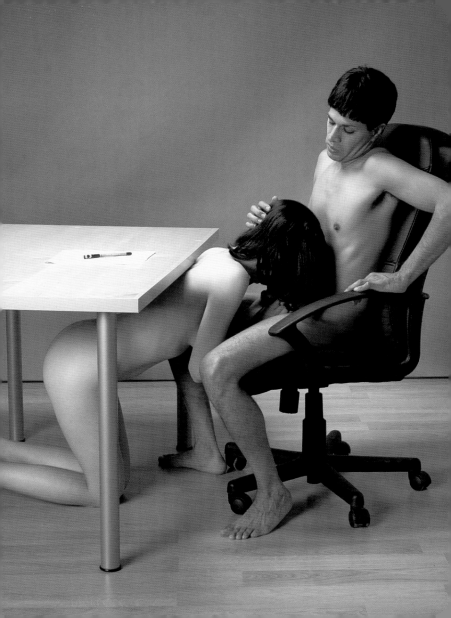

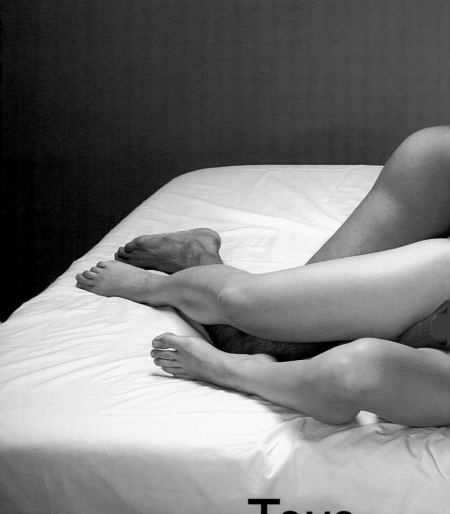

Section Nine: Toys

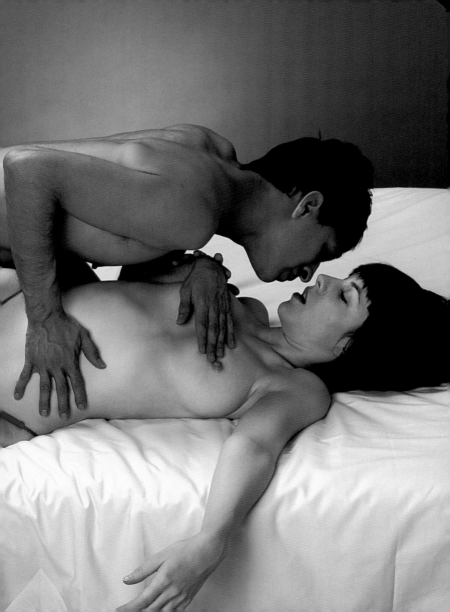

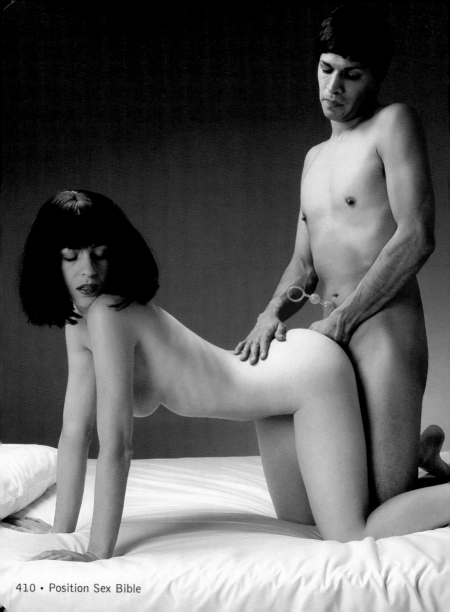

191

Rough Rider

While enjoying See Spot Come (7), the man uses
anal beads to help take her for a wild ride. When
she is ready, he gently inserts the beads one at a
time, using a lubricant if needed. As she is cli-
maxing, he slowly removes the beads, intensifying
the experience.

192

Performance Art

Better than canvas, the lovers paint
strokes of pleasure onto each other
using body paint and their moans to
guide their inspiration.

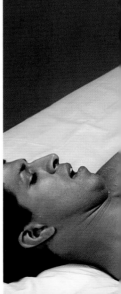

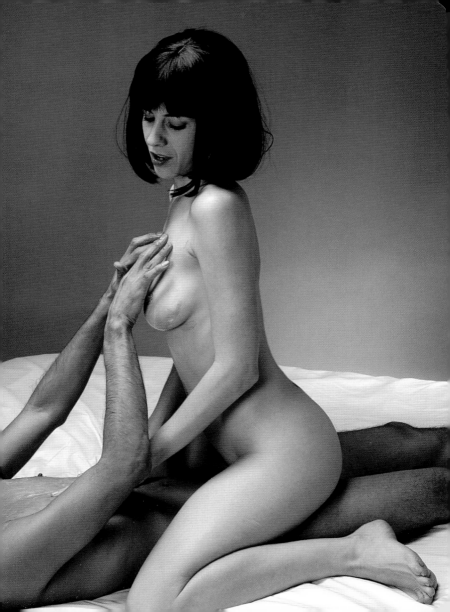

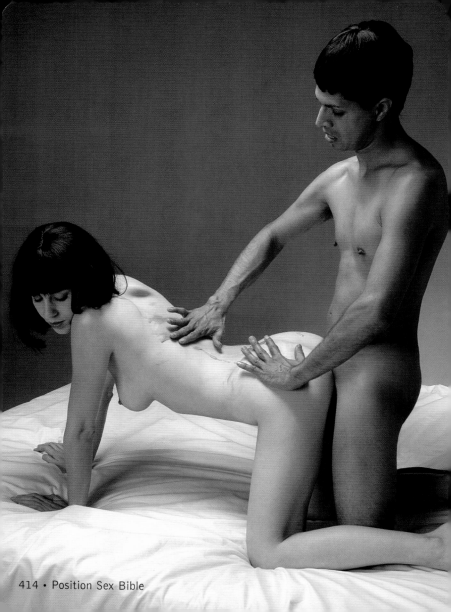

193

Smear Tactics

He enters her from behind, drawing sensuous
patterns with body paint where she cannot
see. He leaves his mark inside and out.

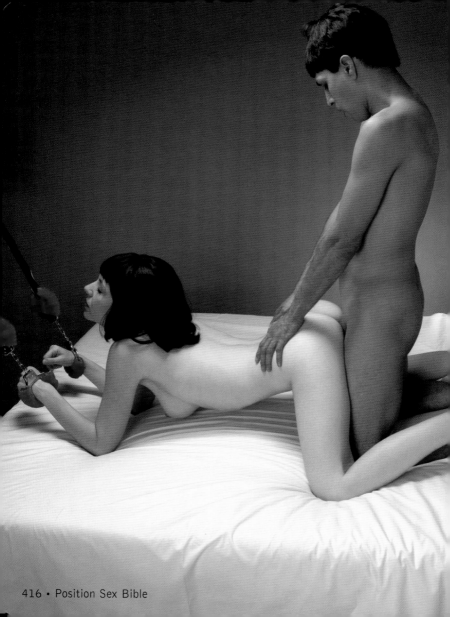

194

Prisoner of Love

His passion (and handcuffs) keep the woman available to her lover's every whim. He chooses to take her from behind, holding her firmly, telling her he's in charge.

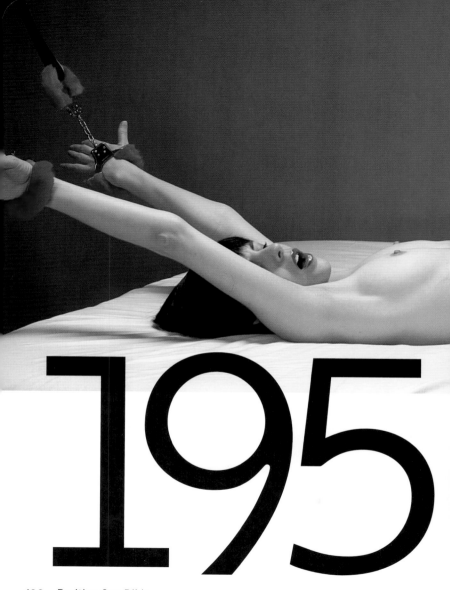

195

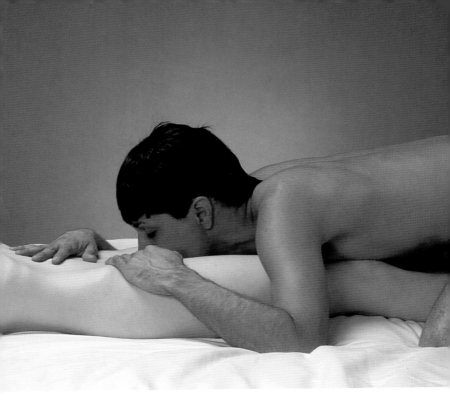

Love Slave

(or the Benevolent Dictator)

Power has its privileges and responsibilities. The helpless
woman, tied to the bed with love and ropes accepts her lover's
munificence as he shows his appreciation for her loyalty.

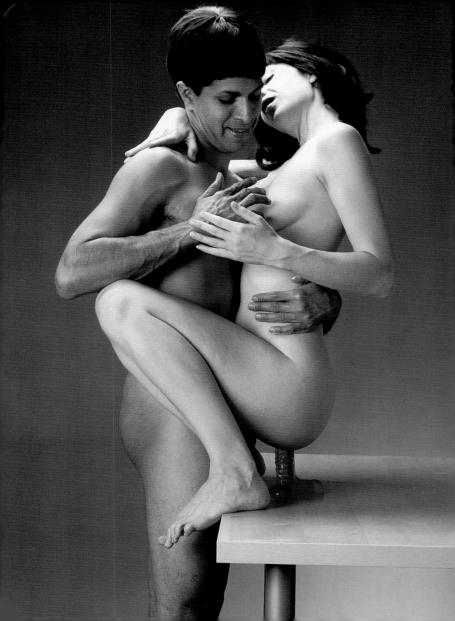

196

Impaled Passion

The suction-cup dildo stays in place on the table as the woman moves up and down on it. Ah, the wonders of science. She presses close against her lover allowing his living equipment to rub against her. He adds to the mix by caressing her breasts.

197

Working Every Angle

She's draped over an ottoman. He uses a vibrator to tease and touch her vagina and clitoris. He uses a hand to tickle her anus. She grabs at the floor in pleasure.

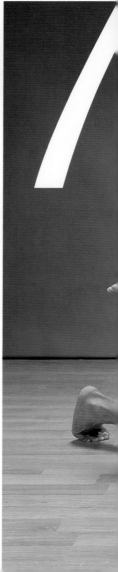

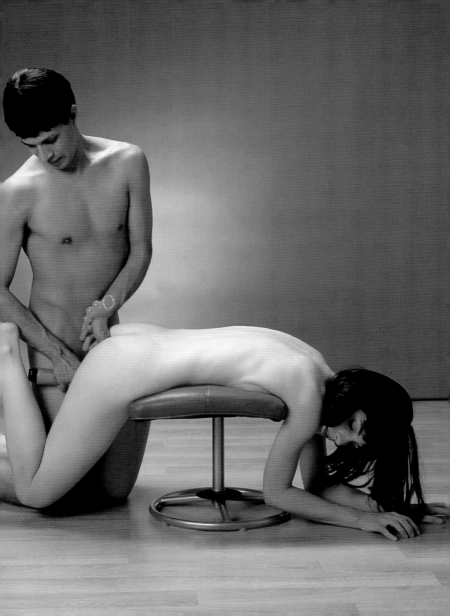

198

Trapped Bumblebee

A pair of tight panties holds a vibrator snuggly in just the right spot. The man can then make the other parts of the woman's body buzz with his mouth and hands.

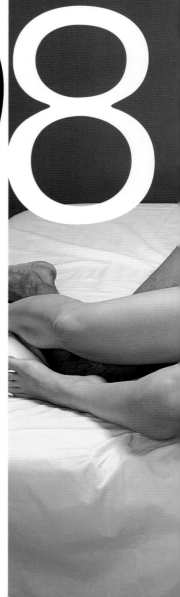

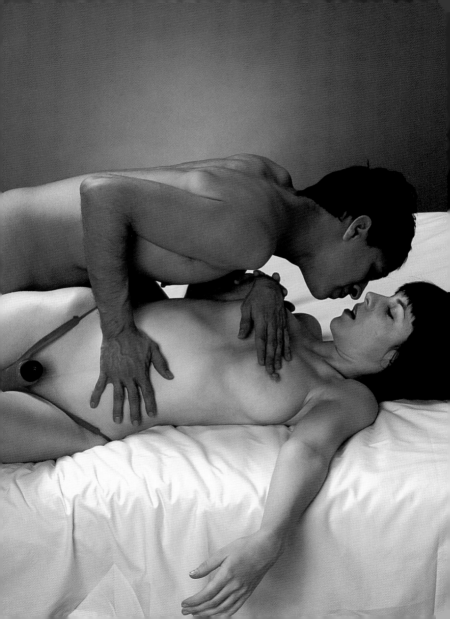

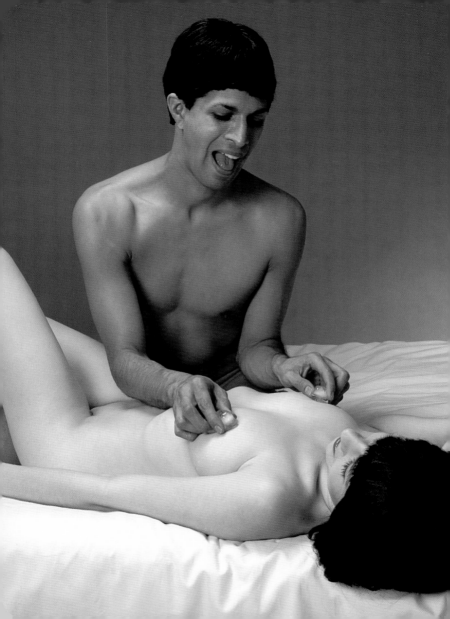

199

Fire and Ice

The ice is cool, his mouth is hot. He alternates using both on his lover's nipples. She closes her eyes. Which will it be—fire or ice?

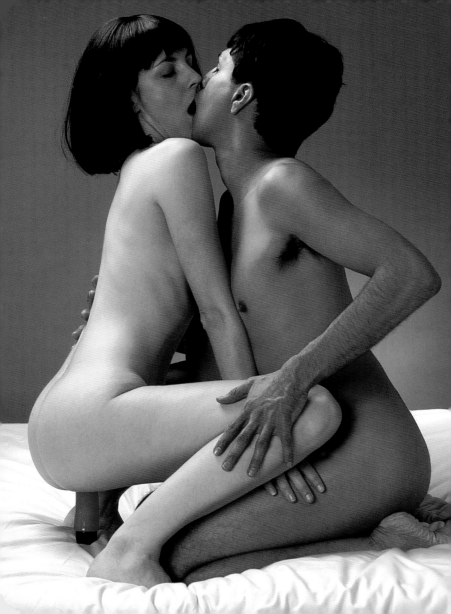

200

The Earthquake

(Butterfly on a Pin)

The man kneels on the bed. His lover squats in front of him. He holds tightly on a vibrator, allowing her to lower herself onto the moving earth.

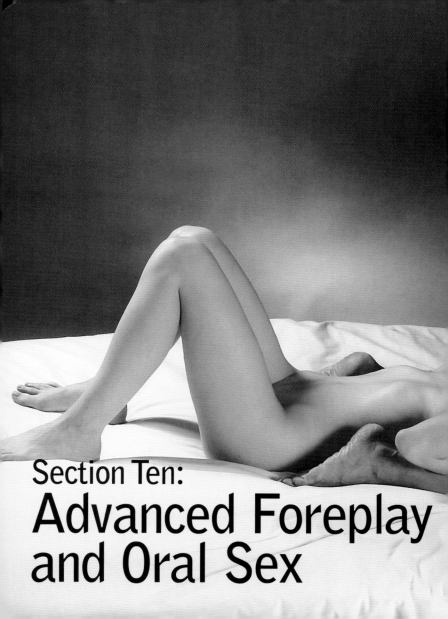

Section Ten:
Advanced Foreplay and Oral Sex

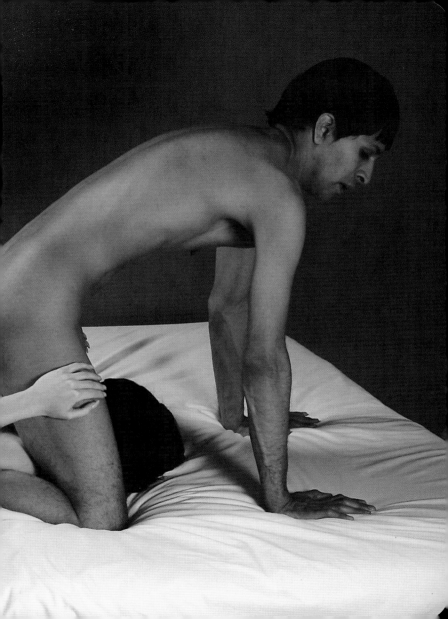

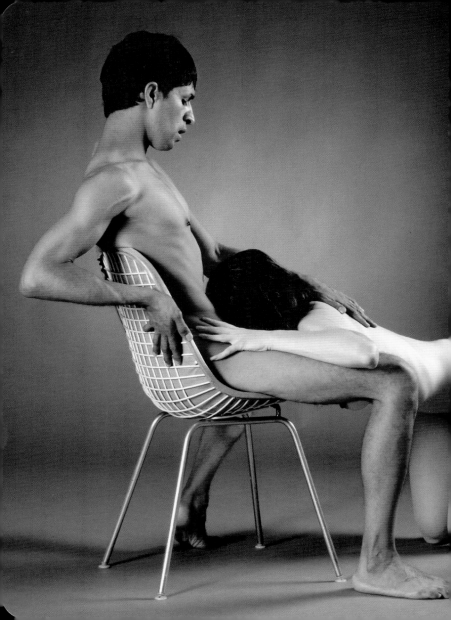

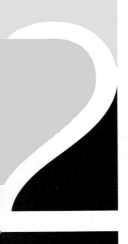
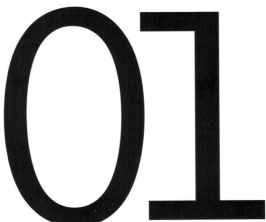

201

The Classic

Sitting down, the man is pleasured orally by the woman, who kneels before him. He is able to enjoy the view from this position of power. His hands are free to caress her head, but this position is focused on him.

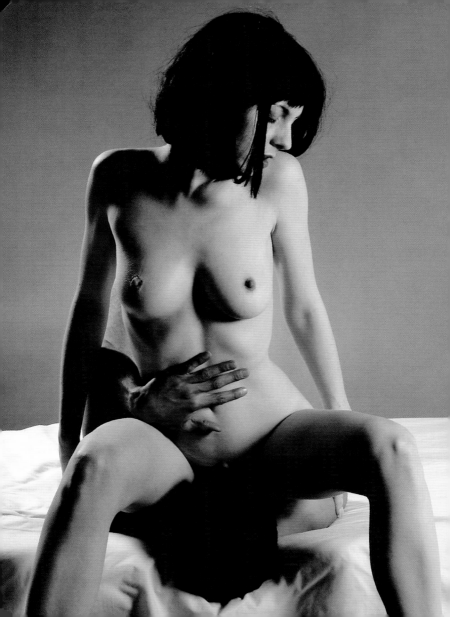

202

Eating In

Allowing the woman full control, the man lies on the bed with his head over the edge. She sits spread above him and straddles his face as he explores her most delicate parts with his lips and tongue, bringing her to climax.

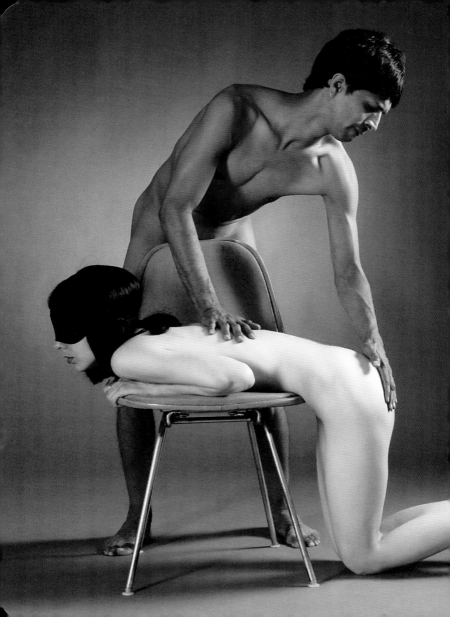

03

Stand and Deliver

He stands behind the chair, and asks, "Yes?"
Wearing a blindfold, she kneels beside the chair
and leans over it, clasping the side of the seat
with both hands and elbows at her side. She
replies, "Yes." He rests one hand on her back,
holding her securely in place as he firmly slaps
her buttocks before gently tickling her anus.

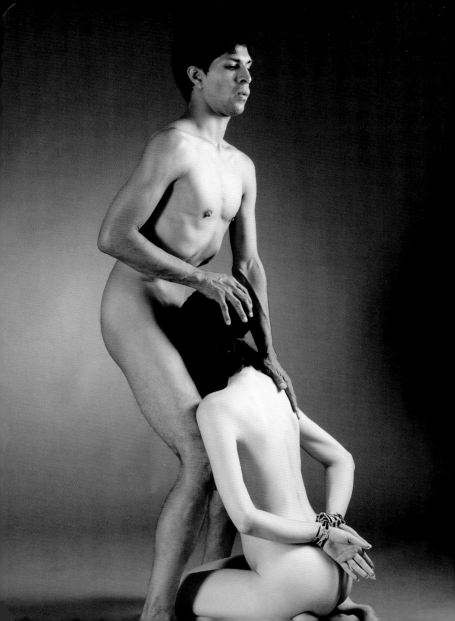

204

Nose to the Grindstone

Still blindfolded, she kneels on the floor and sits
on her feet with her hands tied securely behind
her back. Holding her shoulder, he bends his
knees slightly and guides her head to lick and
suck his testicles and penis.

205

Take It Sitting Down

The woman sits before the man and pleasures him with her mouth. More comfortable for the giver than the typical kneeling position, the man receiving fellatio here will appreciate his partner's added attention as he is penetrated anally.

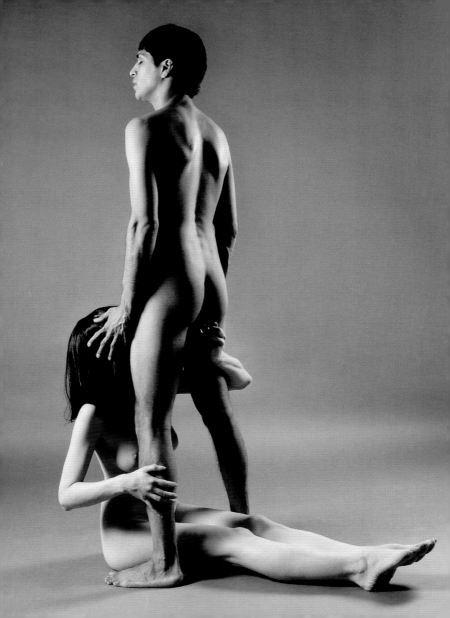

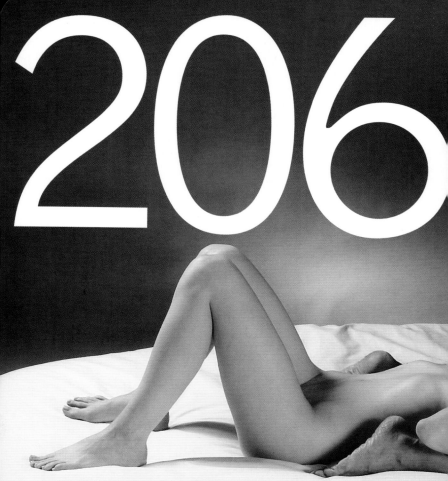

206

The Happy Puppy

The woman lies on her back and the man kneels on top of her, doggie style. She is given a full view of him as she takes him into her mouth, leaving a hand free to massage his testicles or finger his anus.

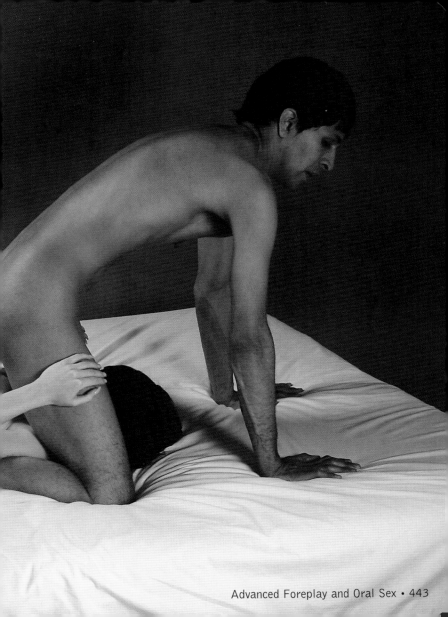

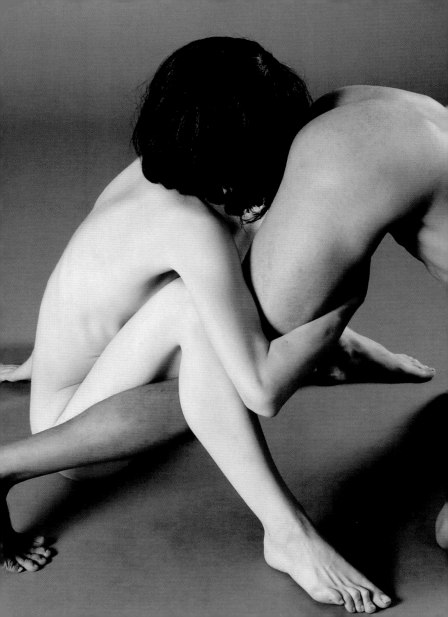

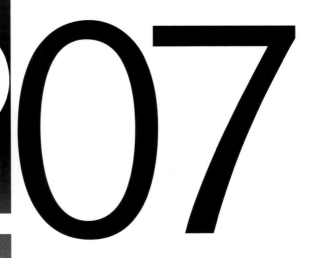

207

The Ben Dover

As the man bends over, he opens himself up for her tongue to stimulate his anus. She uses her free hands to touch his penis, giving him two pleasures for the price of one.

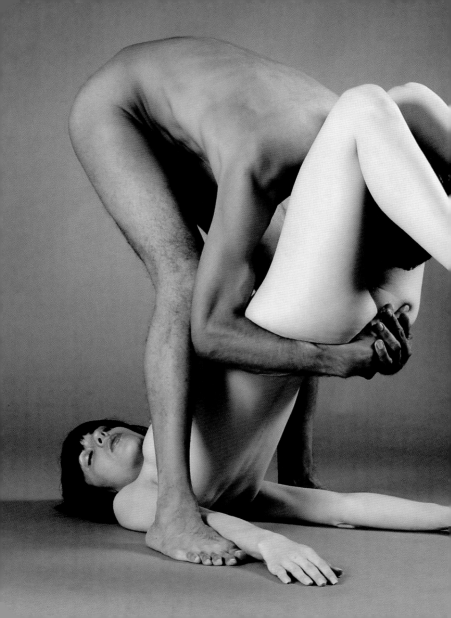

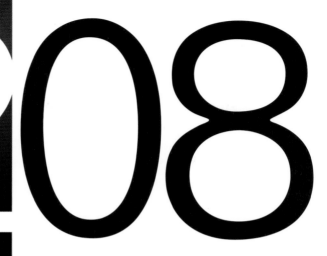

208

The Circle of Pleasure

The woman lies on the floor and is lifted by the man, who bends slightly over her to pleasure her with his tongue. She is able to return the favor by touching him with her two free hands.

209

Kiss My . . .

As the woman stands with her bottom slightly out, the man sits and pleasures her with his mouth. She can keep her hands on the back of his head, and control the depth of his tongue. From this position, the woman can fantasize that anyone, including her partner, is behind her, making her come.

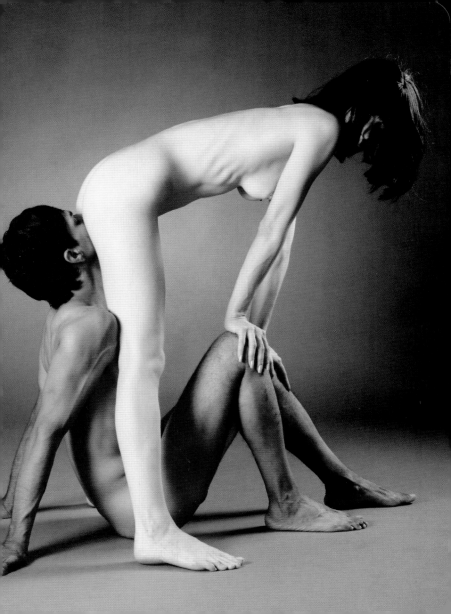

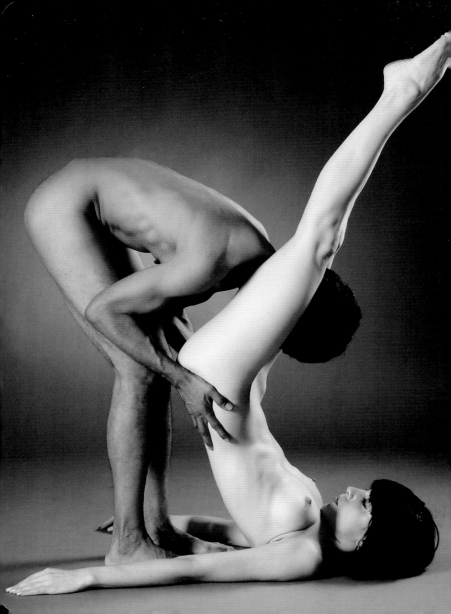

210

The Elevator

She raises her legs and balances on her shoulders
as he bends down to perform cunnilingus on her,
supporting her back and stomach. This can easily be
modified for multi-partner sex, but we'll leave that
to your imagination.

211

The Landscape of Two Mountains

The man lies on his back with knees bent as the woman straddles his face, leaning her weight on his chest. He proceeds to provide oral sex while lifting her up with his hands on her behind, giving himself room to breathe.

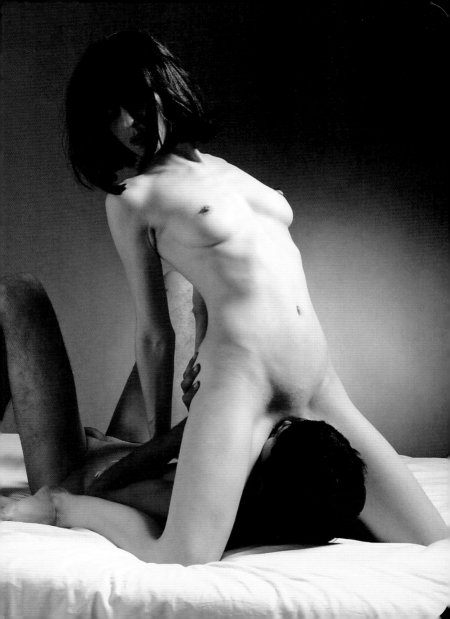

212

The Curled 69

The man and woman perform oral sex on each other simultaneously, but curl into a tucked position to create a tighter, more intimate position as they cradle each other into orgasm.

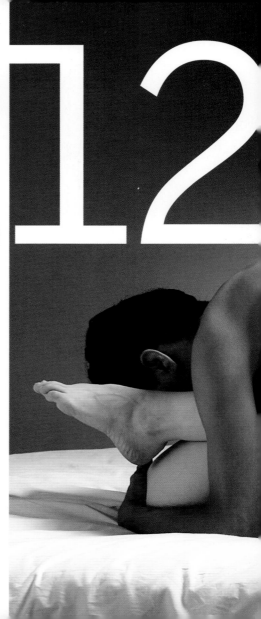

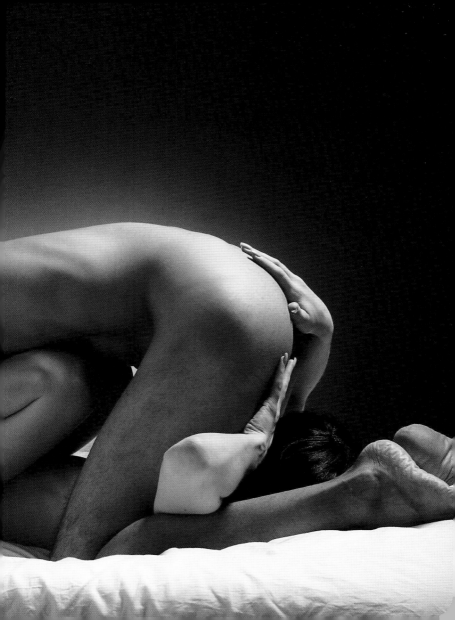

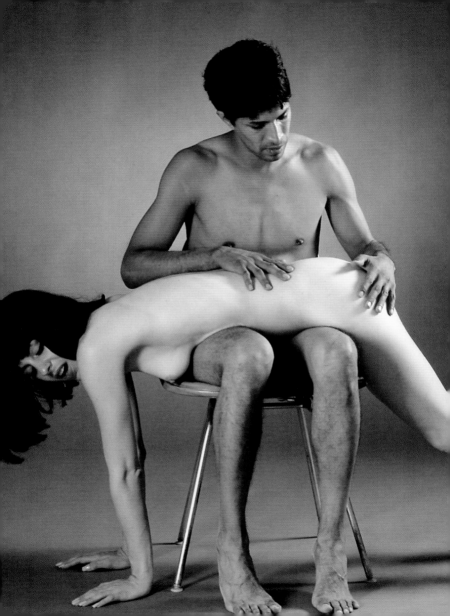

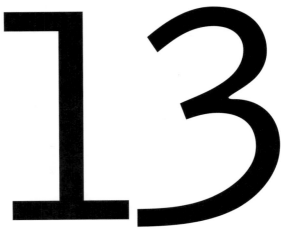

213

Slap and Tickle

The man sits in a chair with the woman standing beside him. She stretches herself over his lap, supporting herself on her hands and the tips of her toes. He holds her by pressing the lower half of his arm to keep her firmly in place, while he spanks and strokes her buttocks, making her bottom red, tingly, and hot.

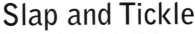

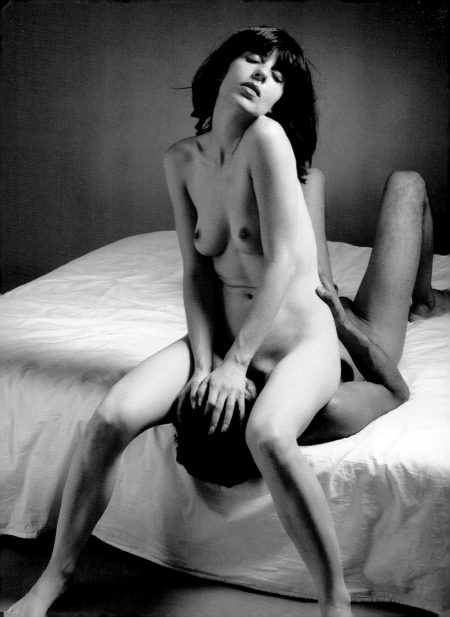

214

Oh, Adam, What an Apple

The man lies face up so that his head is at or near the edge of the bed; the woman straddles his face, keeping her feet on the floor and lowers her vagina to his mouth. He can use his hands to stimulate her clit and her anus.

215

Give Him a Hand

The reversal of the Slap and Tickle, the man extends himself over the lap of his partner and is spanked repeatedly, turning his bottom a pleasurable shade of apple red.

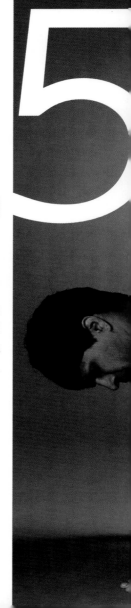

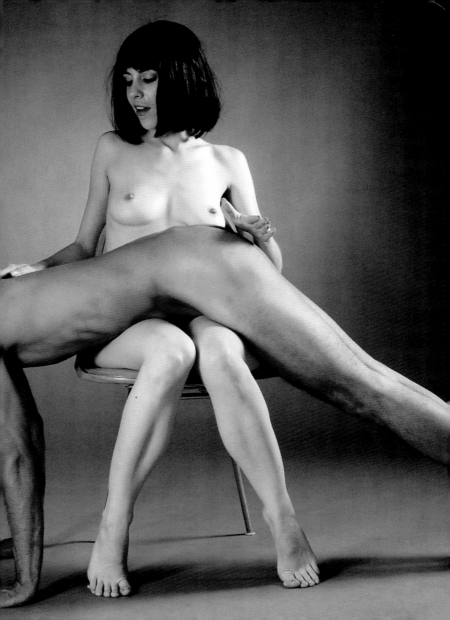

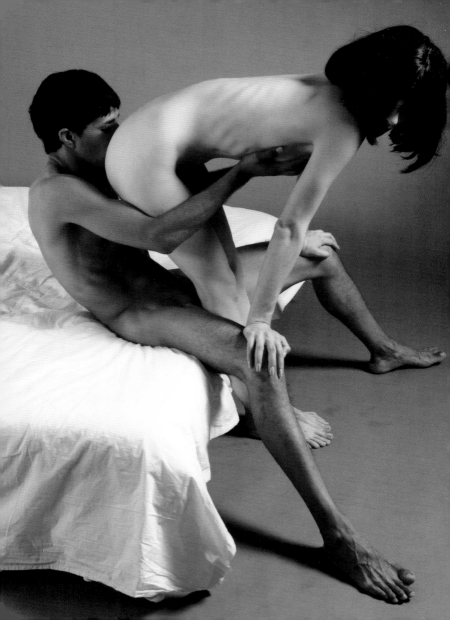

216

0 Marks the Spot

He leans on the edge of the bed and straddles his partner, who is bent before him. He licks her anus and fingers her clitoris and nipples, stimulating several erogenous zones at once to create a powerful orgasm.

217

Mistress May I?

Blindfolded, the man crouches on the floor
with his hands secured around him with his
tie. The woman stands before him and, cup-
ping her hands around his head, guides his
mouth to her nether regions and instructs
him to do precisely what she desires.

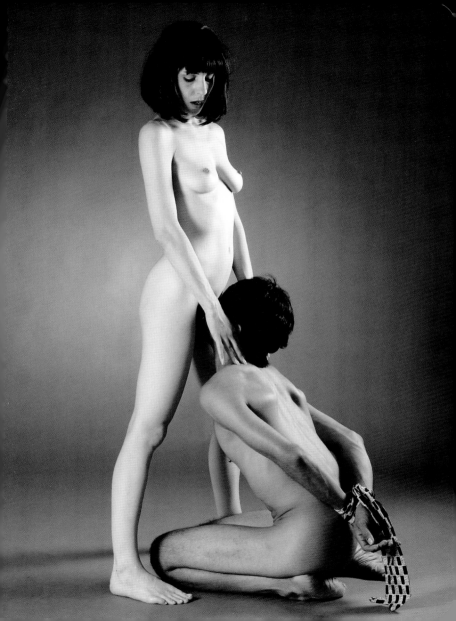

218

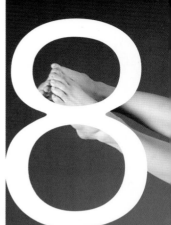

The Sack of Potatoes

As the man lifts the woman by her hip and turns her slightly, she stimulates his penis with one hand, while caressing his body with the other.

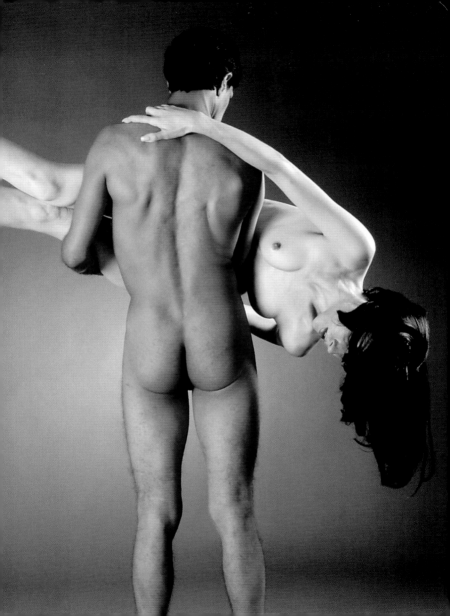

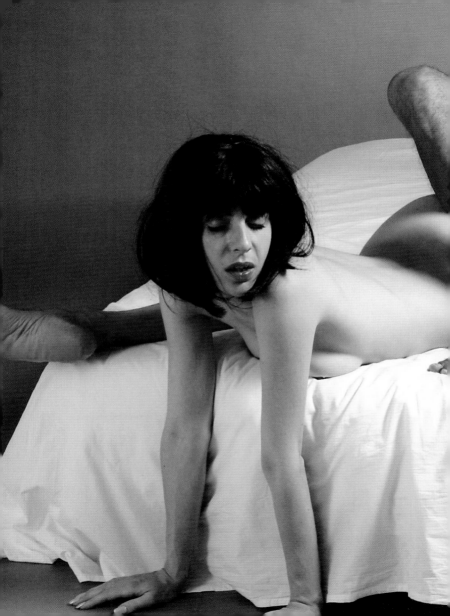

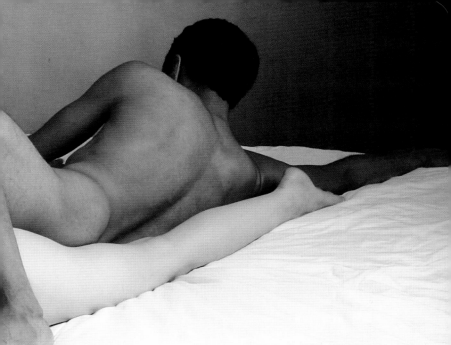

Section Eleven:
Taking It to Another Level

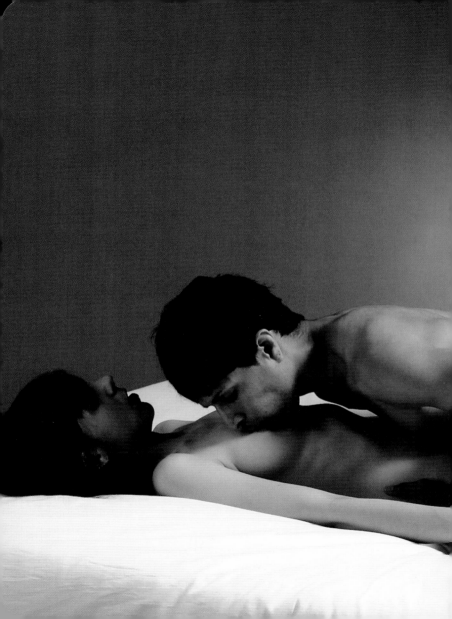

219

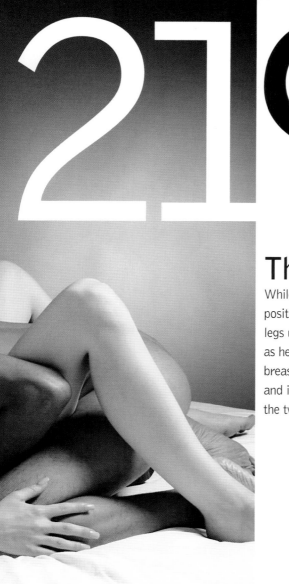

The Cradle

While in the missionary position, the man brings his legs up to cradle his partner, as he slowly kisses her breasts, creating a sensual and intimate moment for the two.

220

Hammocking

Squatting to form a chair, the man takes the woman onto his lap, rocking back and forth on the balls of his feet. The woman might want to take control and rock—letting their bodies fall where they may.

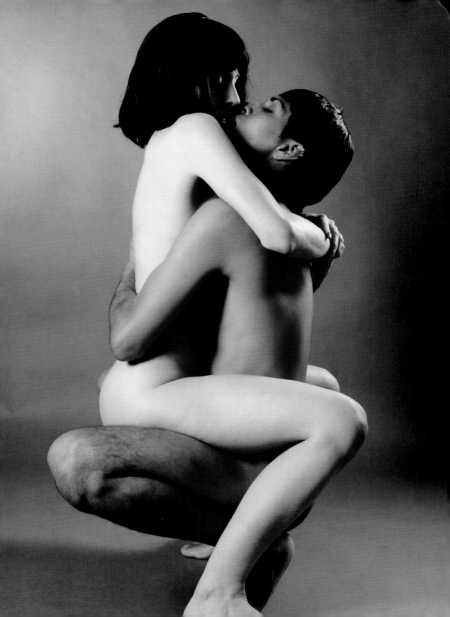

Salted or Unsalted?

The man spreads his legs horizontally and enters the woman, who opens her legs in the opposite direction. She leans back and grasps his leg for support as she orgasms in this delicious pretzel of pleasure.

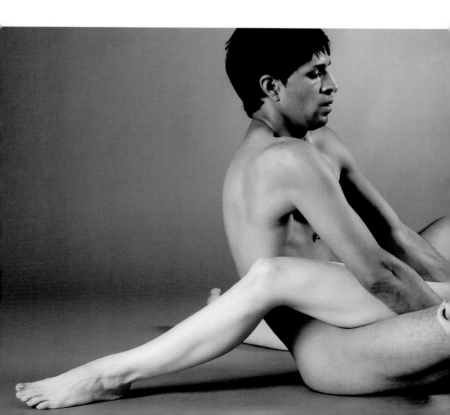

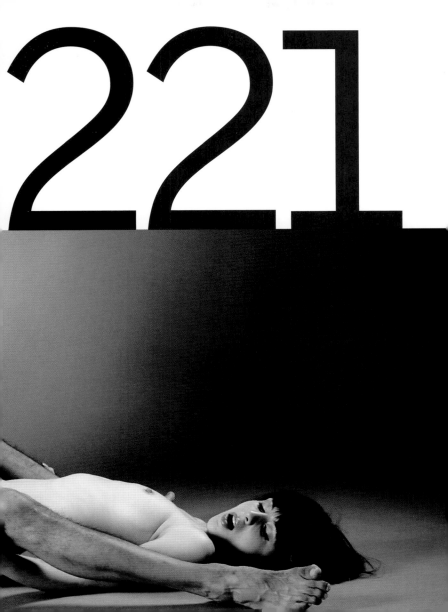

222

Learning to Walk

She lies on her back on the bed with her feet
resting on the floor. He straddles her, facing away
from her and enters her upside-down and hanging off
the bed, using his arms for balance. She wraps her
left leg around his back and to his right shoulder.

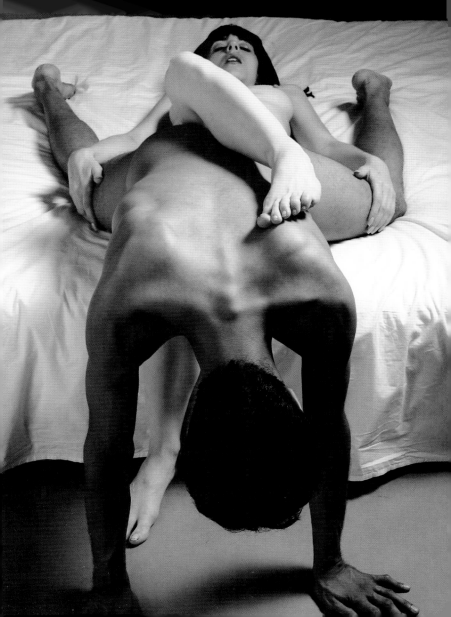

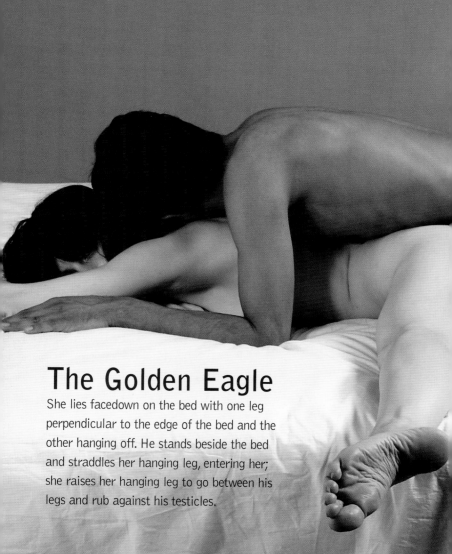

The Golden Eagle

She lies facedown on the bed with one leg
perpendicular to the edge of the bed and the
other hanging off. He stands beside the bed
and straddles her hanging leg, entering her;
she raises her hanging leg to go between his
legs and rub against his testicles.

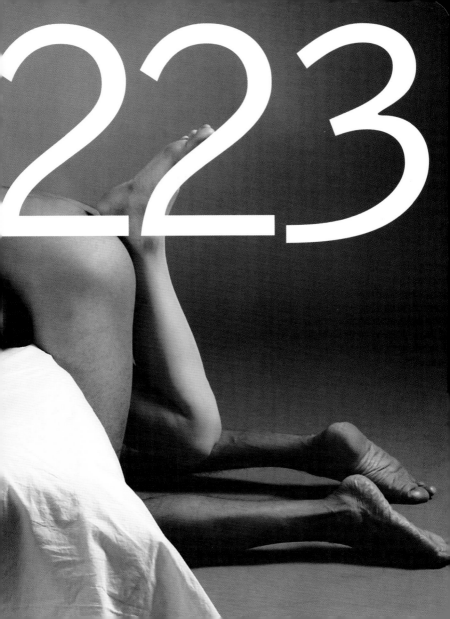

Crossing the River

The man enters the woman from behind, arching his back and allowing her to imagine her deepest fantasies. He supports her with his leg, and the couple creates a bridge to paradise.

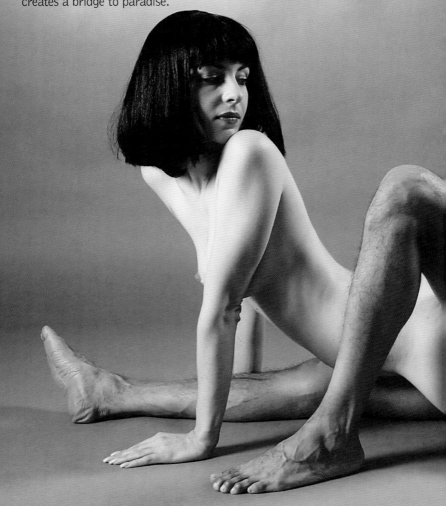

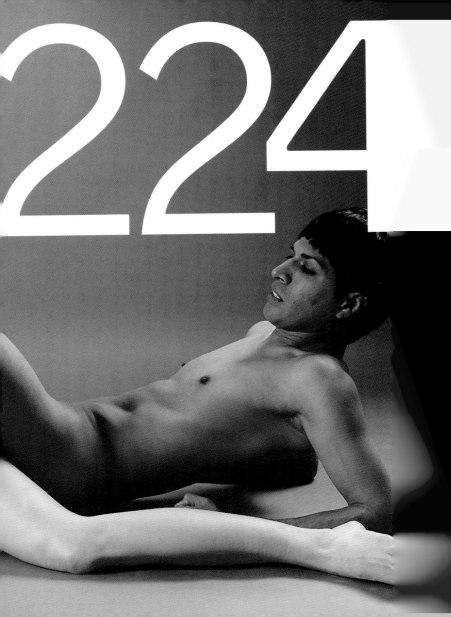

224

The Carriage House

She gets down on all fours, allowing him to kneel down and enter her from below. He now leans back and watches as she slides back and forth.

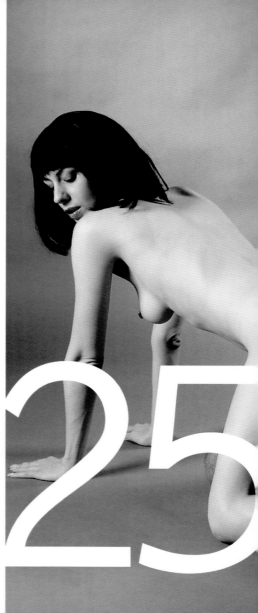

225

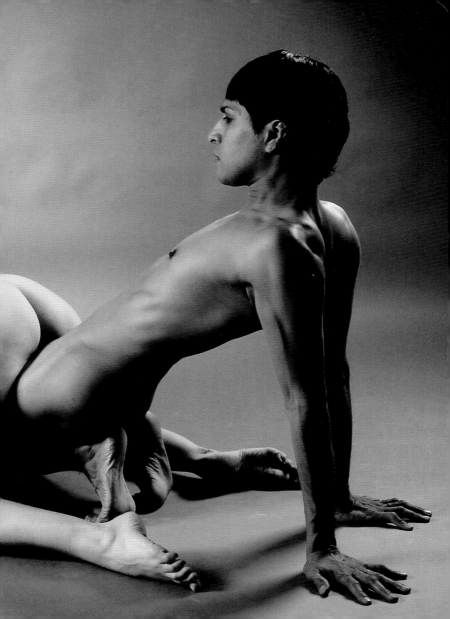

226

Catch You on the Flip Side

He lies face up on the bed, and facing away from him, she straddles him, bending her knees behind her, leaning back on her hands and sliding down to mount him. He loosely grazes his hands around her hips, helping her to pace her strokes.

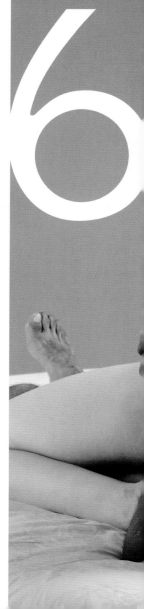

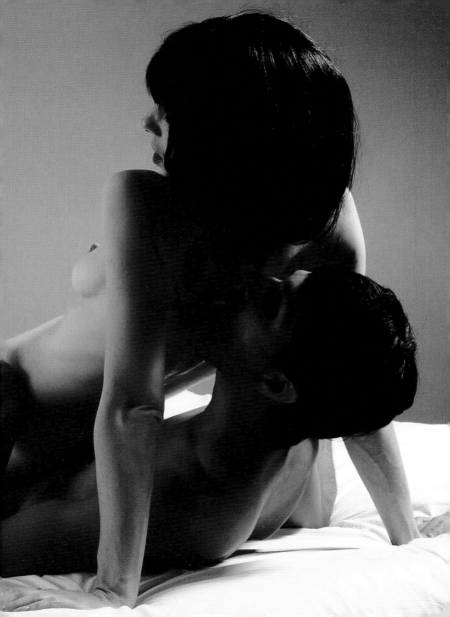

227

The Intertwined Links

Lying on their sides, head to toe, the couple merge their private parts. She may now kiss his feet or massage his testicles, while he should feel free to caress her buttocks and thighs.

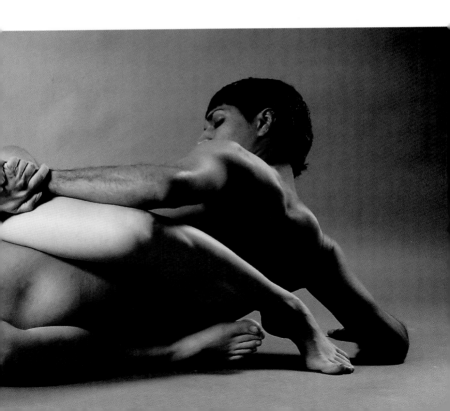

Chain Me Up

Lying on the floor with his legs in a V, the man enters the woman anally while she bridges over him, creating a chain link. This position requires effort, but is well worth it.

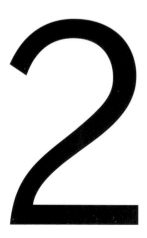

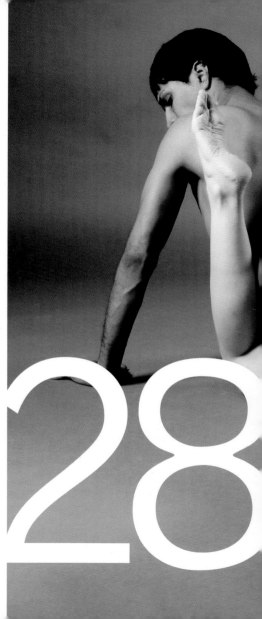

228

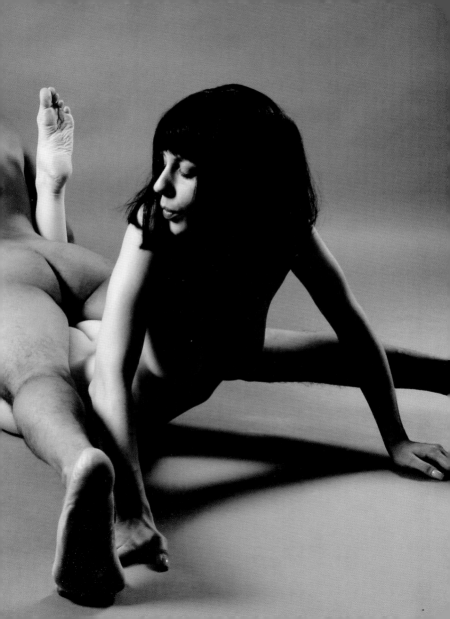

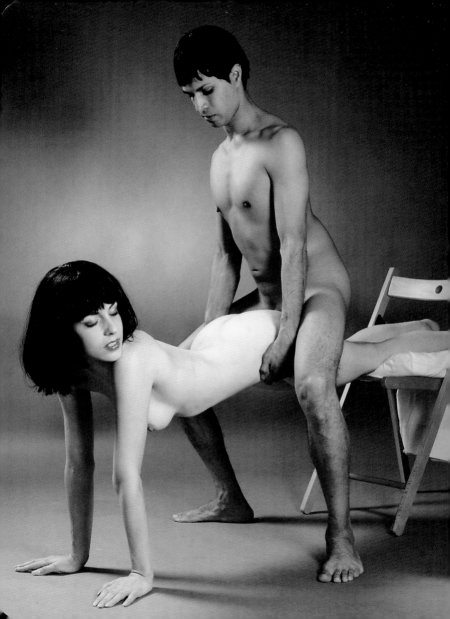

229

Shucking the Oyster

She rests her legs on the chair while keeping her weight on her arms as he enters her from behind and caresses her body with his hands.

230

Under Wraps

The man sits on a chair and wraps his legs around his partner's waist, as she supports him from below. She takes the lead and decides when and how deep to thrust.

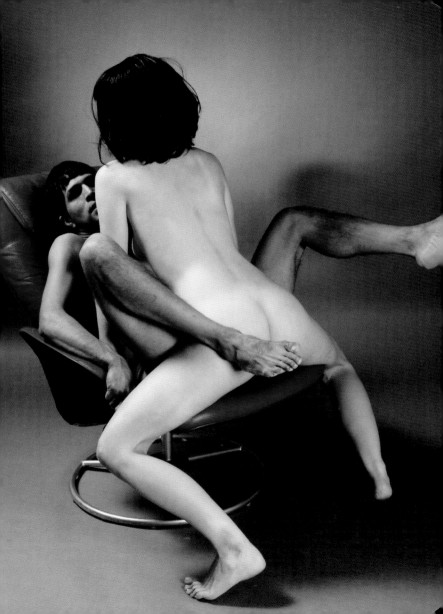

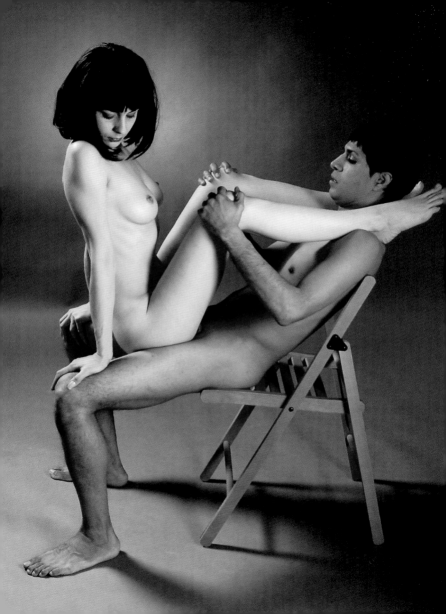

231

The Kitchen Sink

She sits on his lap and balances herself with her hands on his thighs, squeezing as she orgasms. He is free to watch himself penetrate, as she spreads her legs over his shoulders.

232

Rock-a-Bye Baby

As he sits on a chair, she straddles him and leans forward as they clasp hands for support. If he is on a rocking chair, he might rock slowly, while he is afforded a beautiful view of her from behind, and she is rewarded with a feeling of flying.

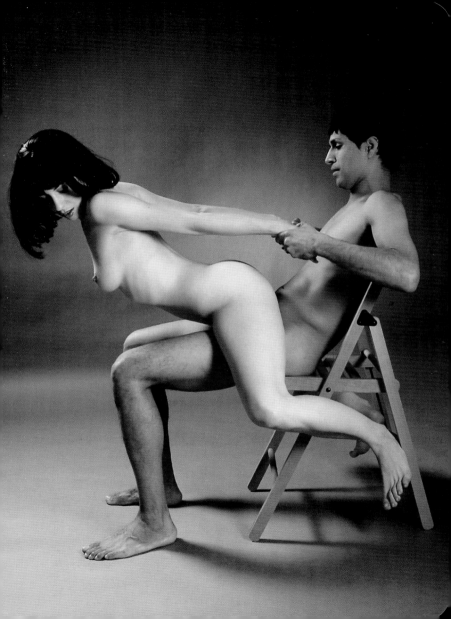

233

The Curling Iron

The woman rests her torso on a rocking chair, and he enters her perpendicularly as she curls her legs around him. She can easily stimulate her clitoris, and he is free to stroke her whole body.

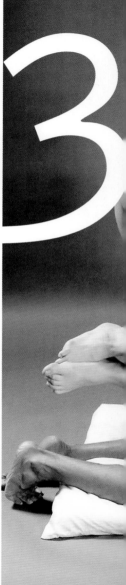

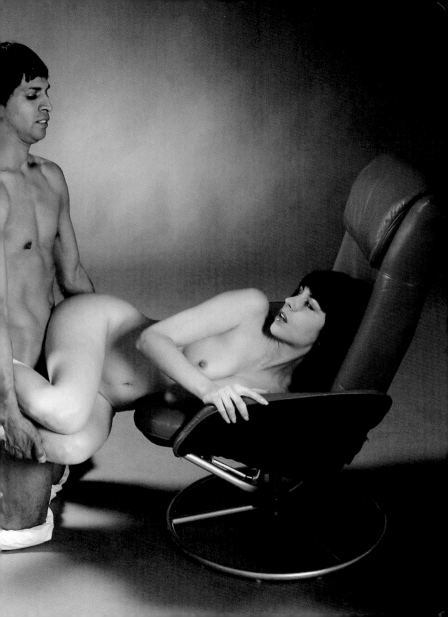

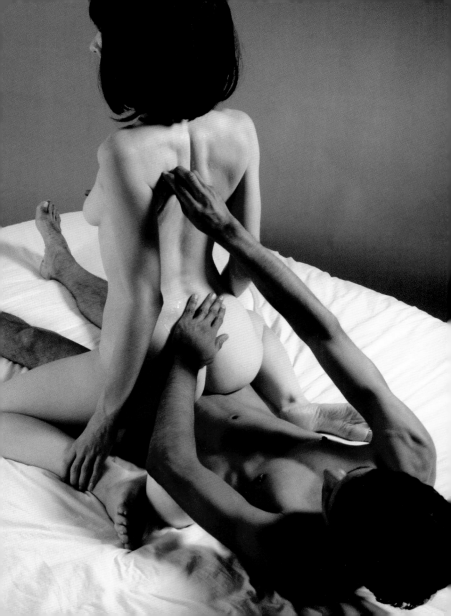

234

Like a Cat

He lies on the bed on his back, and she straddles him facing his feet, with her back arched. He rubs ice on her buttocks and back, cooling her kittenish heat.

235

On the Road

He bridges on his shoulders as she squats above him, grabbing one of his calves and pulling it forward, controlling his movement with as much precision as she would handle a standard shift automobile.

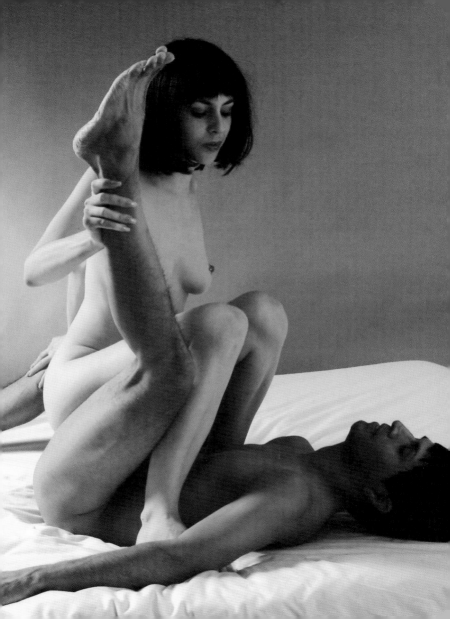

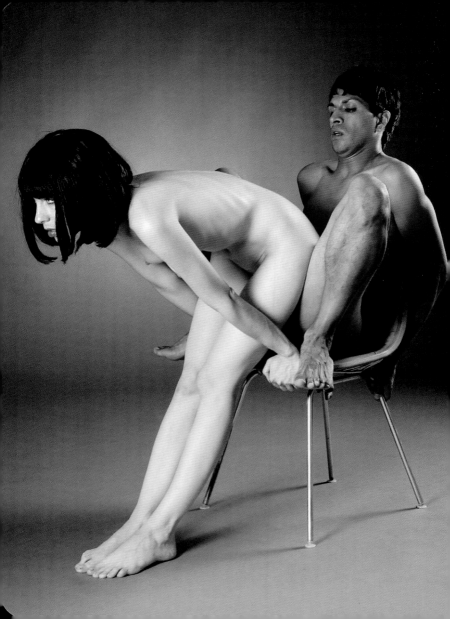

236

The Whoopie Cushion

Grasping the back of the chair, the man lifts himself up and balances on the seat on the balls of his feet, entering the woman, who stands before him, from behind. She holds the legs of the chair for extra support and balance.

237

Sailor's Knots

The man sits in a rocking chair as the woman leans down opposite him, raising her legs to rest behind his head. He rocks them back and forth while penetrating. This position can be reversed, and the woman is free to stimulate the man's prostate while taking the lead.

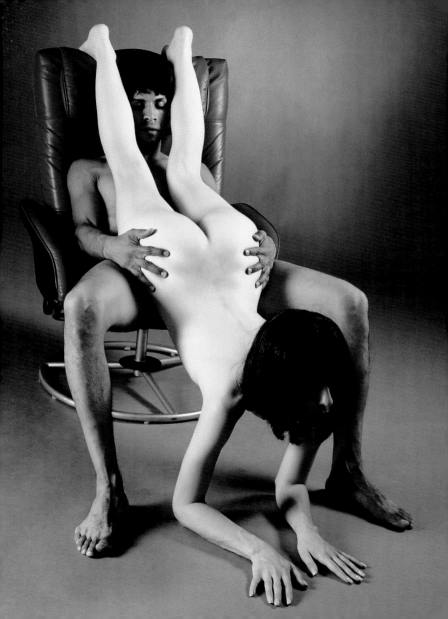

238

The Cancan Dancer

The woman raises one leg and rests it on the chair while she is penetrated from behind. Her hands are free to grab his thighs to pull him deeper into her, and his are free to caress her body.

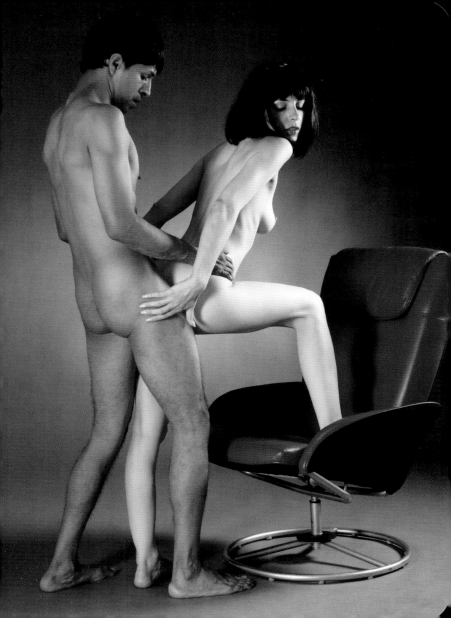

239

The Venus Flytrap

The man lies back on an ottoman, lifting his bent legs, and takes the woman onto himself as she leans back into him. She can grasp onto his legs and caress his feet to increase his sensations.

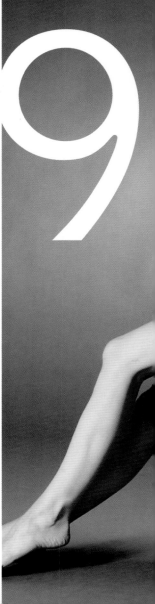

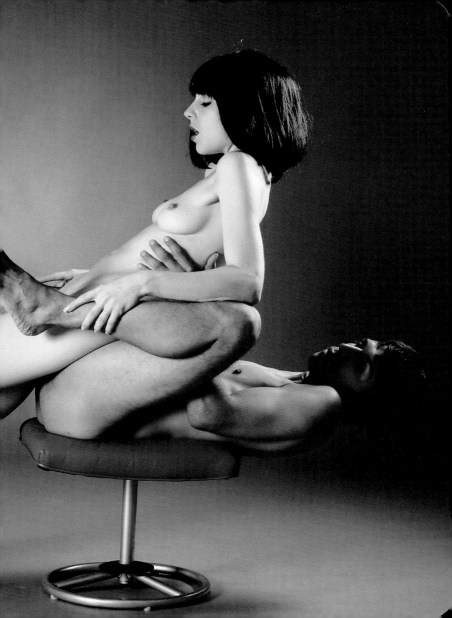

240

The Homestretch

Resting his head on the chair, the man supports himself with his hands, and enters the woman, who holds her legs back and open as far as they'll go while lying on the ottoman. This stretch is a good preparation for the Three-Chair Double Squat (241).

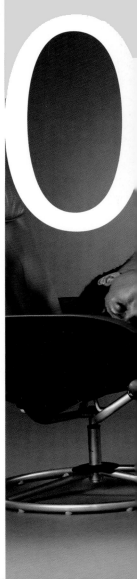

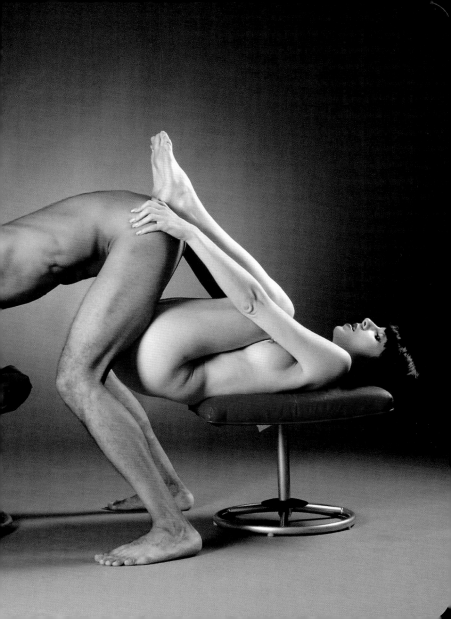

241

The Three-Chair Double Squat

The woman squats between the man's legs, which he has spread open and supported by a chair each, as he leans back on the ottoman, supporting himself with his hands.

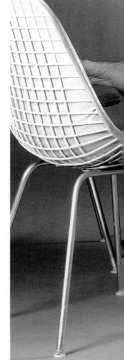

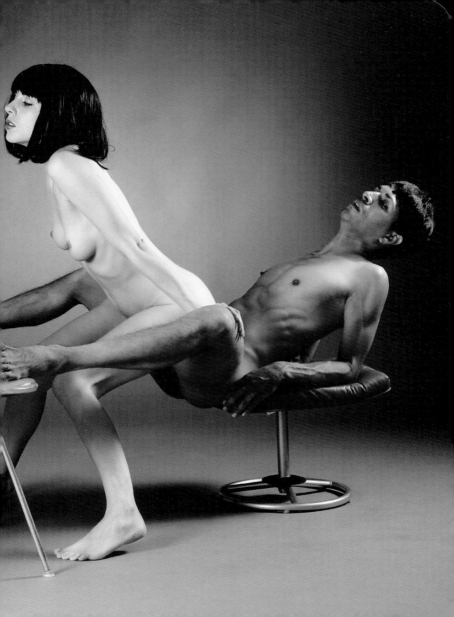

242

Doing Cartwheels

The man lies on his back and lifts his legs in a split. The woman then sits between his legs, allowing him to enter her. From this position, she is able to control every movement.

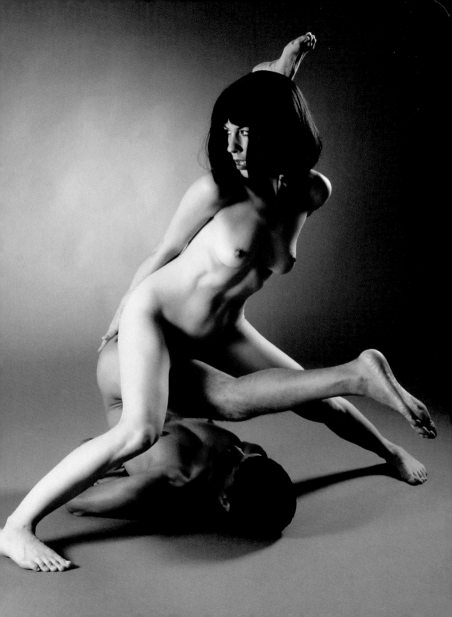

243

The Headstand of Pleasure

As the woman lies on the floor, the man lifts her so that she is parallel to him, supporting herself with her shoulders. They grasp behind each other's knees, an erogenous zone, and support each other this way.

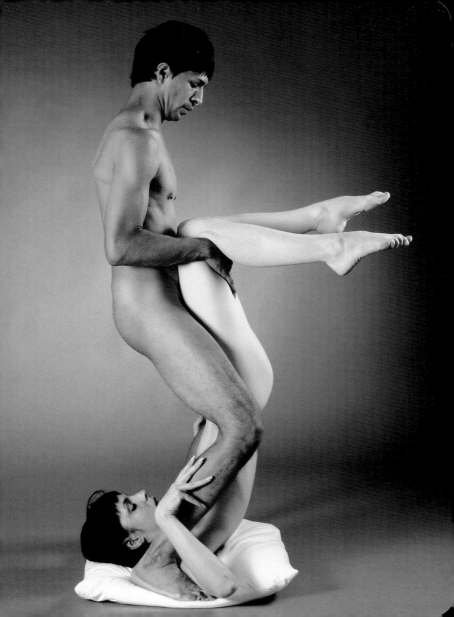

244

Pole Vaulting

The man lifts the woman sideways and enters her as she supports herself with her arms. He grasps her by the thighs and behind, so as to make her feel secure as well as pleasured.

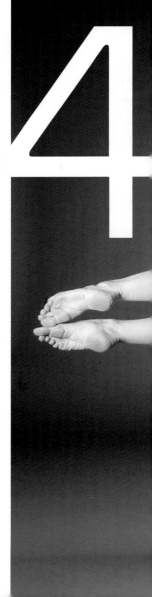

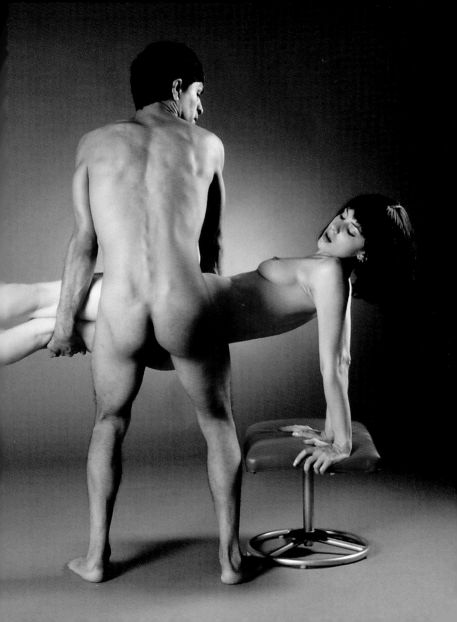

Springing

As he crouches and lifts her legs and torso, she balances herself with her hand behind her head. With her free hand, she can touch herself, providing herself some pleasure and him a show, as he penetrates.

245

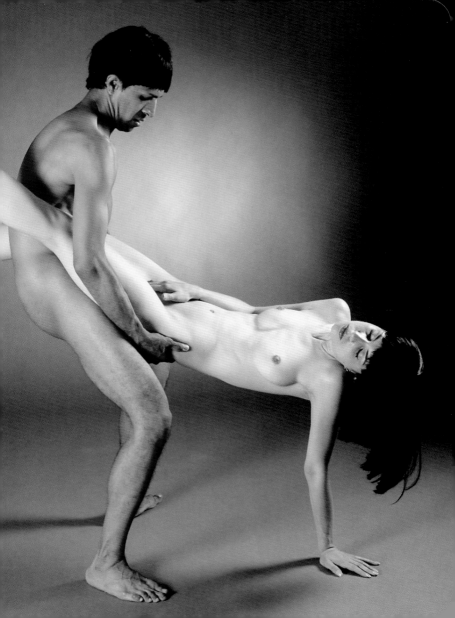

246

The Plow and Hoe

As the man lifts her legs around him, the woman supports herself with her two arms, bridging back in ecstasy. Here he controls the pressure and timing of the thrust as she balances back and enjoys.

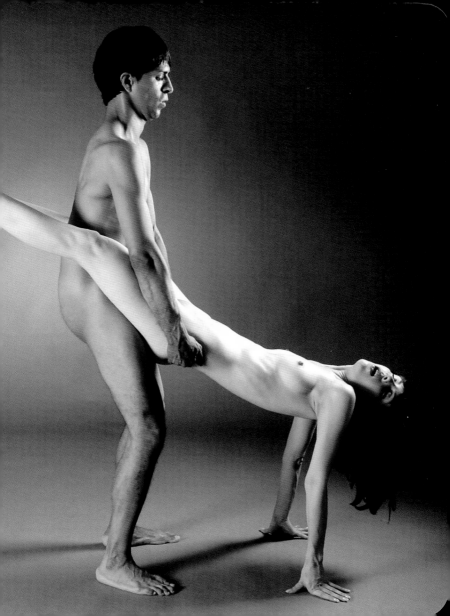

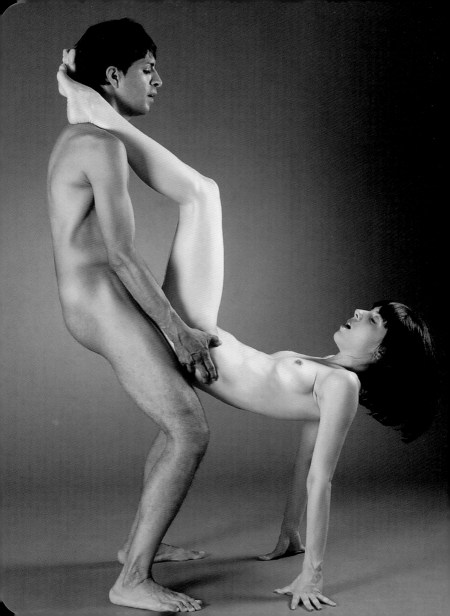

247

Roll Your Rs

The woman balances on her hands as she leans against the man, putting her feet on his shoulders. He grabs her behind, supporting her while providing a pleasurable massage to her bottom, as she roars with rapture.

That's a Wrap

Curled up on the floor, the man enters the woman wrapped up in
passion and cradling each other in an intimate and trusting position.
The man is free to stimulate the woman's anus orally.

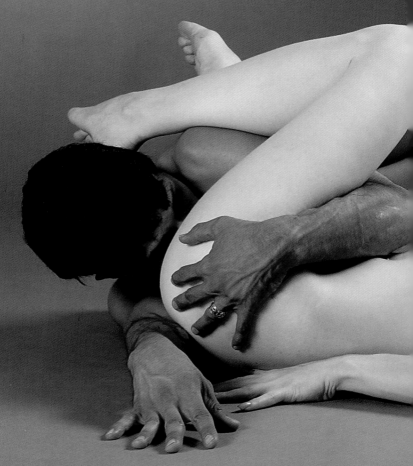

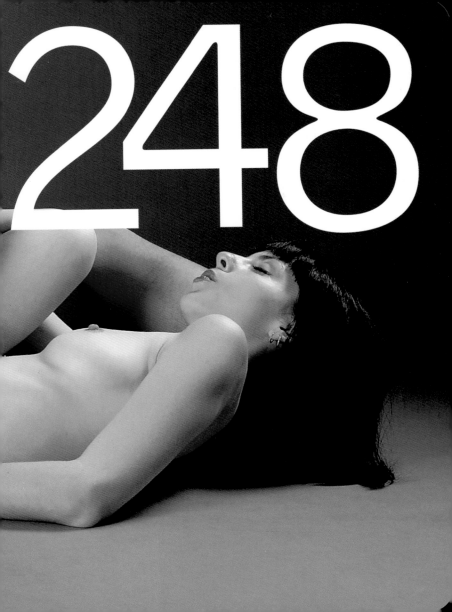

Mountain's Majesty

Facing opposite each other, the man
penetrates the woman from behind
and both raise their legs and
bottoms to create a mountain of bliss.

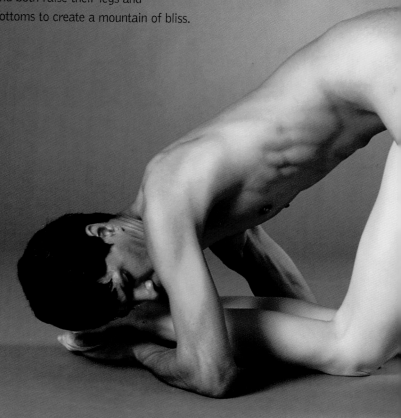

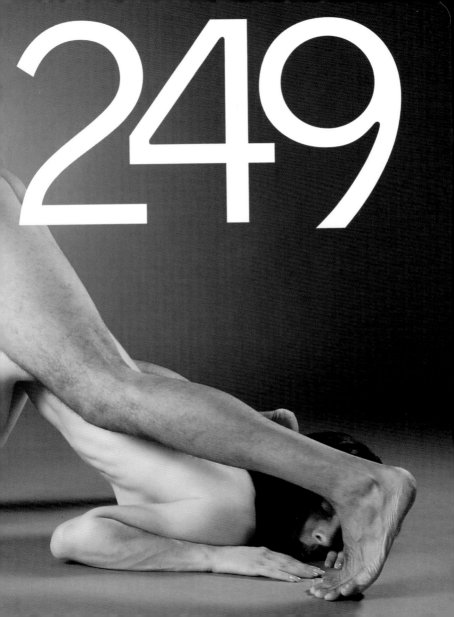

249

250

Crisscross Apple Sauce

He lies on the floor, legs crossed, and she sits on top of him, crossing her legs and stroking his face. The pressure that comes from her crossed legs is sure to give him intense and tight pleasure.

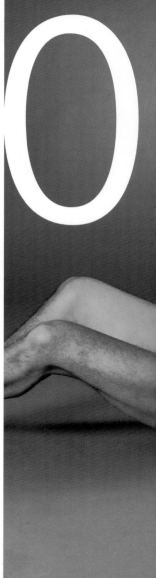

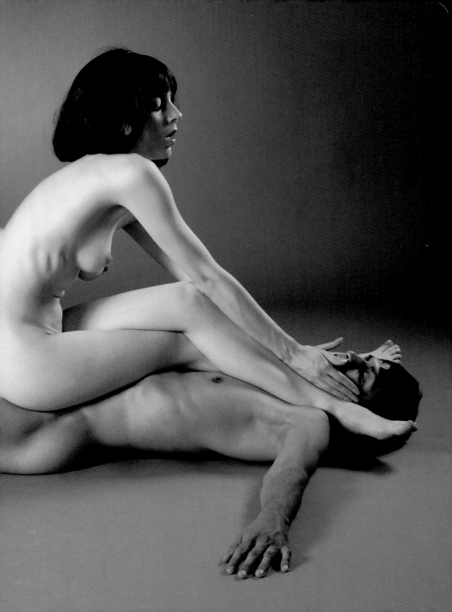

251

Welcome Home

The man kneels and the woman crouches
as she hugs him and he enters her. A highly
intimate position, both partners' hands are
free to explore various erogenous zones.

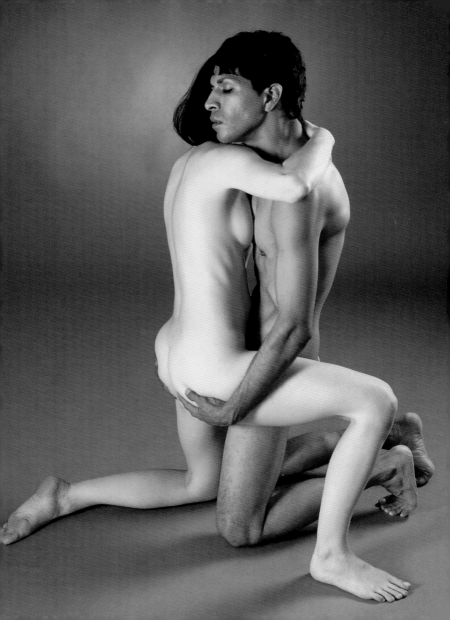

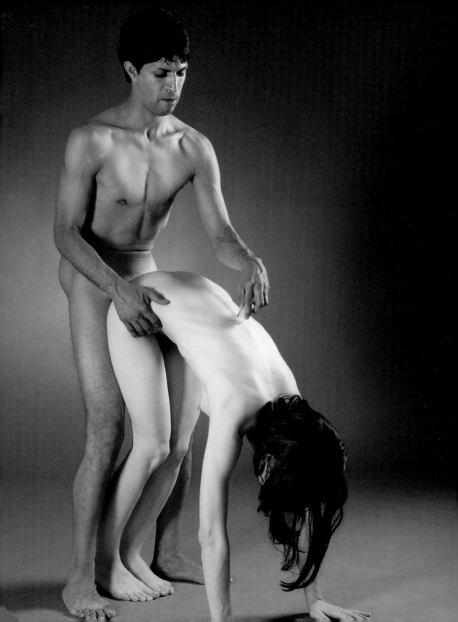

252

Ice Hot

The woman bends in front of the man, who enters her from behind, controlling the rhythm of the act. At just the right moment, he places an ice cube to roam down her back, cooling her heated body.

253

What's for Dessert?

The woman lies on her back and takes the man, who sits between her legs. He holds her torso to maintain a steady thrusting rhythm, while licking chocolate paint from her nipples.

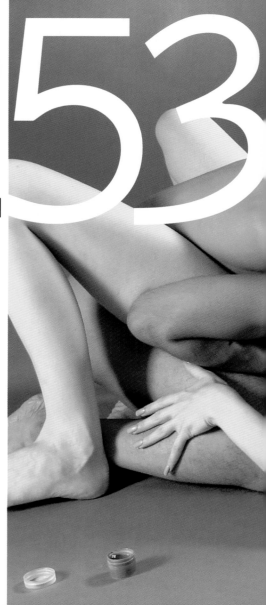

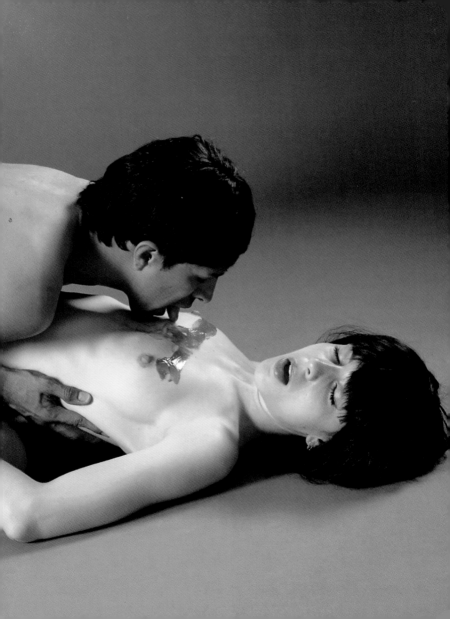

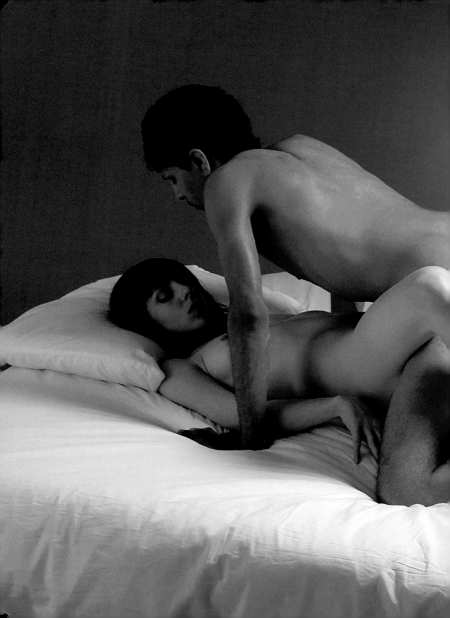

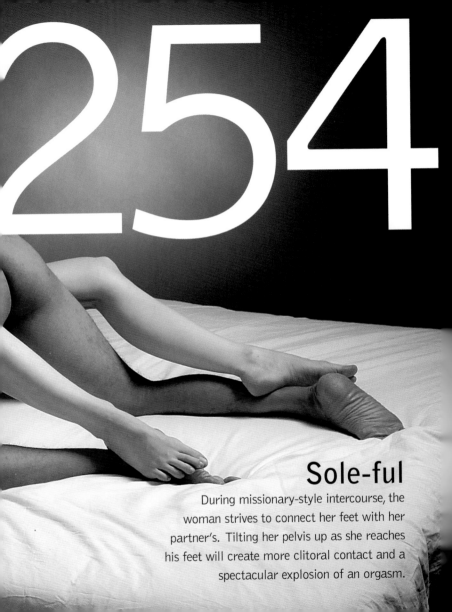

254

Sole-ful

During missionary-style intercourse, the woman strives to connect her feet with her partner's. Tilting her pelvis up as she reaches his feet will create more clitoral contact and a spectacular explosion of an orgasm.

255

Stiletto
High-Rise

Wearing stilettos, she faces the wall, bracing her
hands against it. With her added height, he can easily
enter her from behind while fingering her anus.

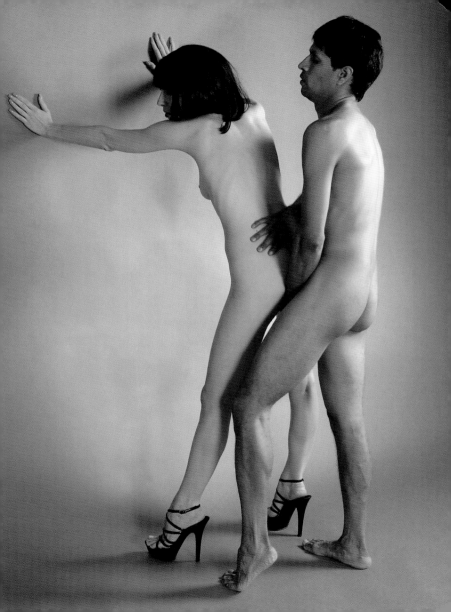

256

See You Later

The woman lies on her back and raises her legs as the man sits facing the same direction and enters her. This leaves him open to fantasies, and renders her capable of scratching or rubbing his back.

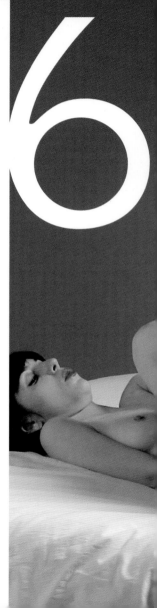

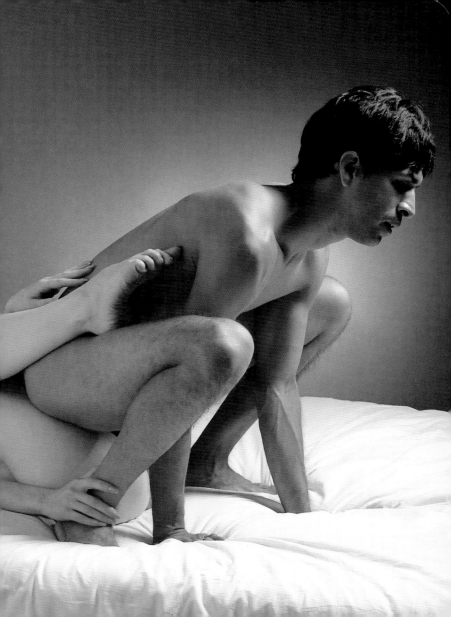

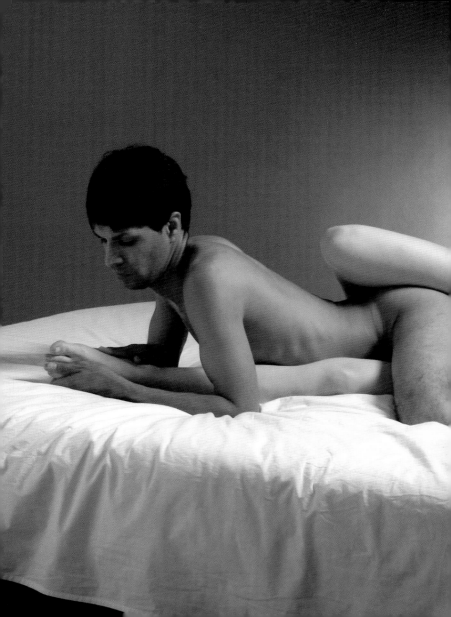

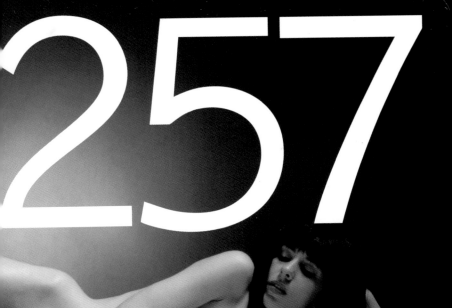

257

The Great Plains

The man enters the woman facing opposite her as her leg is bent to provide ample space for him. He is free to stimulate her feet and enter deeper than ever before, while she can anally stimulate him.

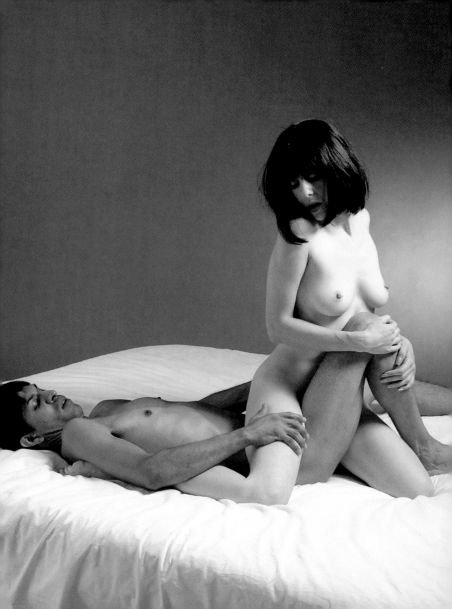

258

For Your Thighs Only

She bonds herself onto his penis and faces sideways and forward so that her clitoris rubs against his raised thigh, creating sizzling friction and an exciting climax.

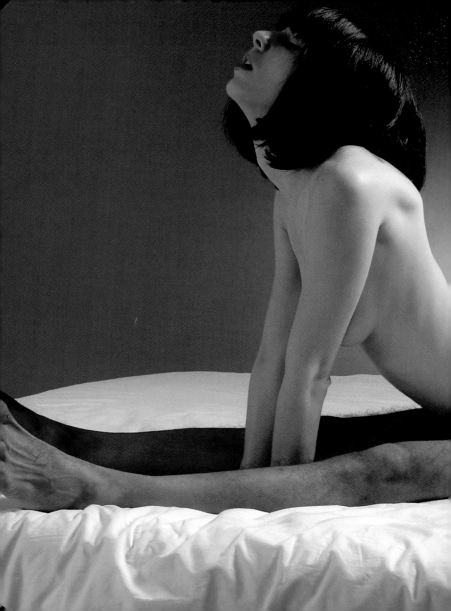

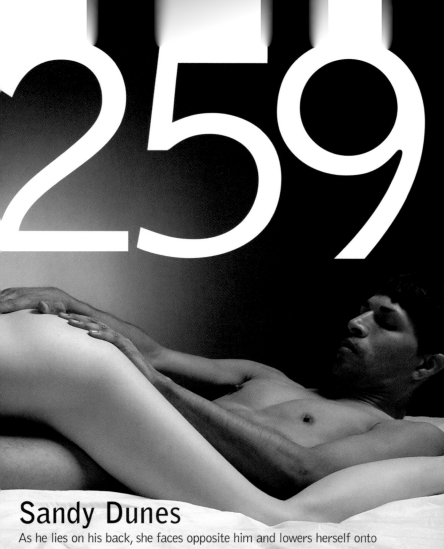

259

Sandy Dunes

As he lies on his back, she faces opposite him and lowers herself onto him. From here, each partner might fantasize about anyone, as well as caress other areas of the body with free hands.

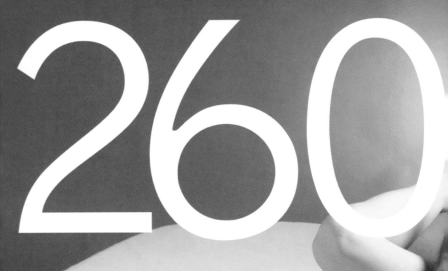

260

Sail Away

She lies on her stomach, and he enters her
from behind, lifting her leg to meet his back,
allowing for deeper penetration and sending
them on a voyage of titanic pleasure.

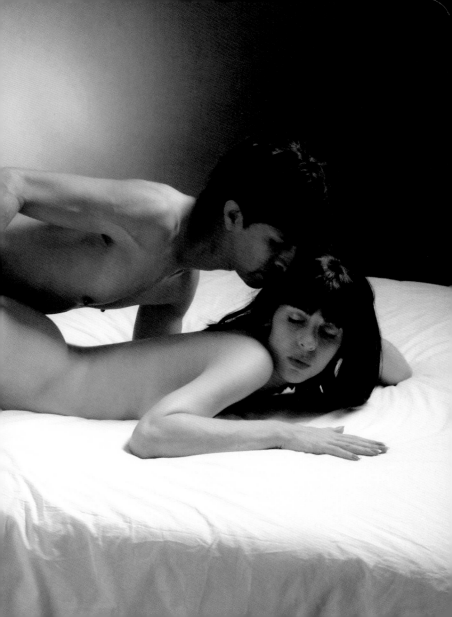

261

The T-Bone

The kneeling man lifts the woman's hips as she lies on the bed in front of him. He enters her from behind, using his free hand to stimulate her clitoris, creating a tender, juicy orgasm, cooked to perfection.

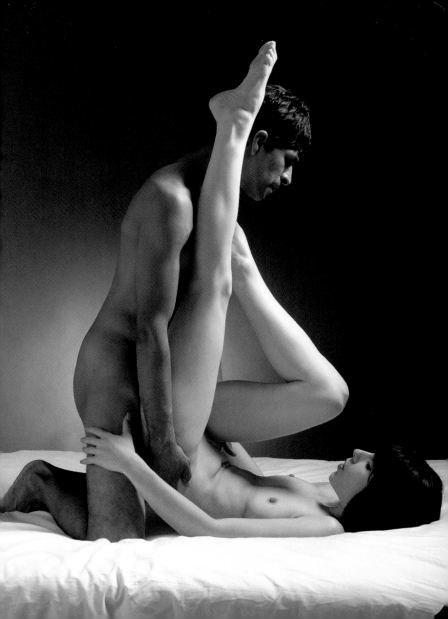

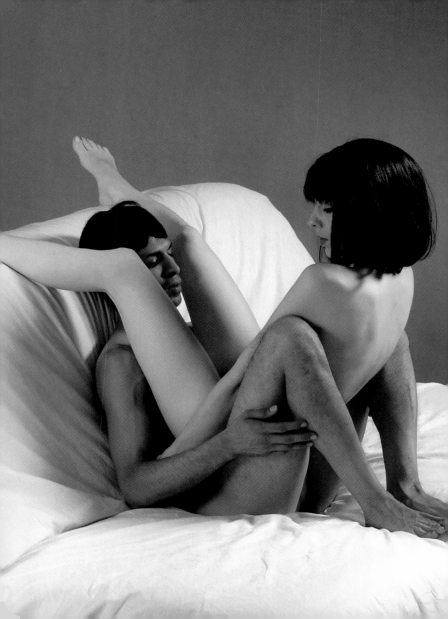

262

Rolling Hills

The man sits in the center of the bed, leaning back on a large cushion with his legs slightly open and his knees bent. The woman lies in the man's lap with her knees falling over his shoulders and her hands gripping his upper arms. He enters her, clasping her waist and rocking their bodies back and forth.

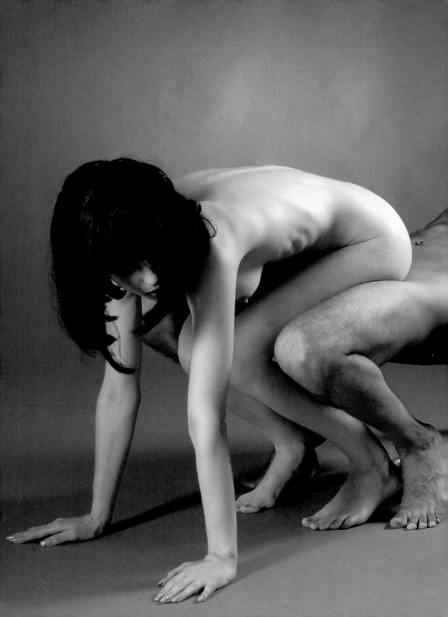

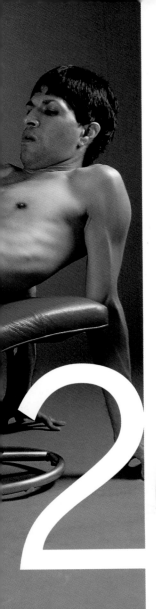

Ready, Set, Go!

The woman crouches on all fours before the man who is seated on the ottoman. He penetrates from behind, leaning back to give her the full length of himself.

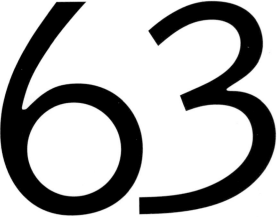

263

The Black Spider

He lies on his back near the edge of the bed and swings his open legs up in the air. Facing away from him, she crouches on her hands and knees on the bed and leans back until their butts are touching. Then she pushes her elbows off the bed until her arms are fully extended and hangs one leg down off the side of the bed. He positions his penis to enter her and then fingers her clit.

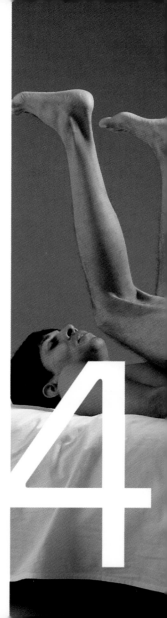

264

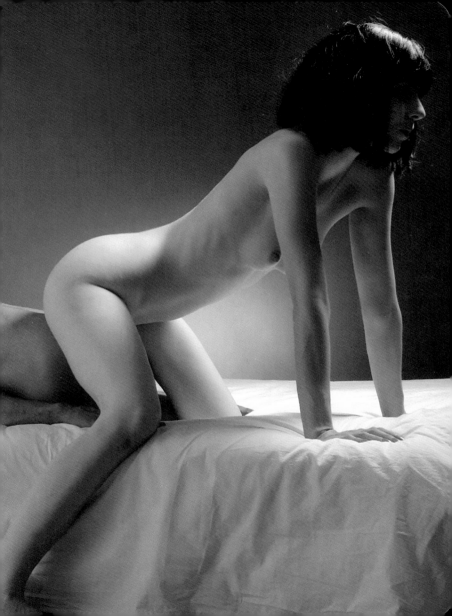

265

The Intimate Hip Grasp

Kneeling on a kitchen chair, the couple can be
adventurous in their setting, but maintain an
intimacy as he enters her from behind and holds
her hips close to his. He is also free to fondle
her breasts and stimulate her clitoris.

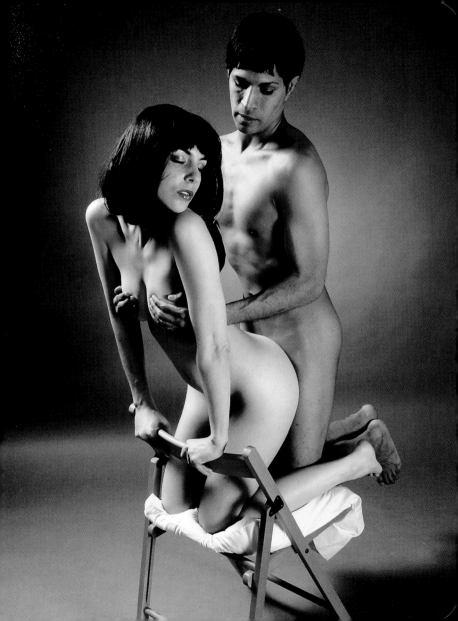

266

Fighter Planes

She lies faceup and parallel to the edge of the bed, with her arms by her sides; he lifts her legs up until they are at a 45-degree angle to her body; then he enters her so that he is perpendicular to her body, supporting his weight with one foot and one arm and raising the others as if flying.

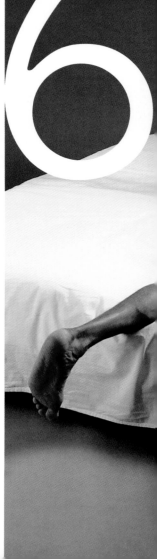

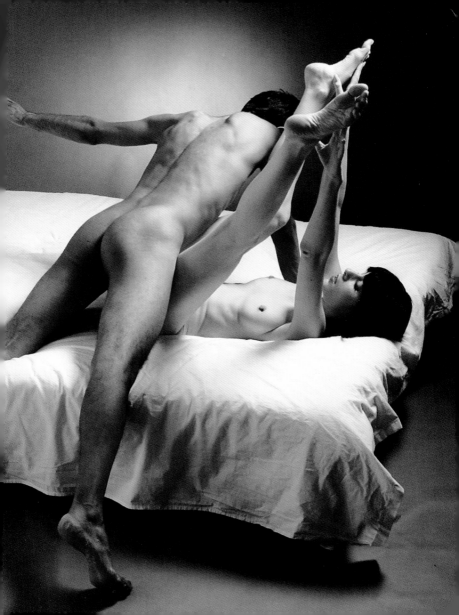

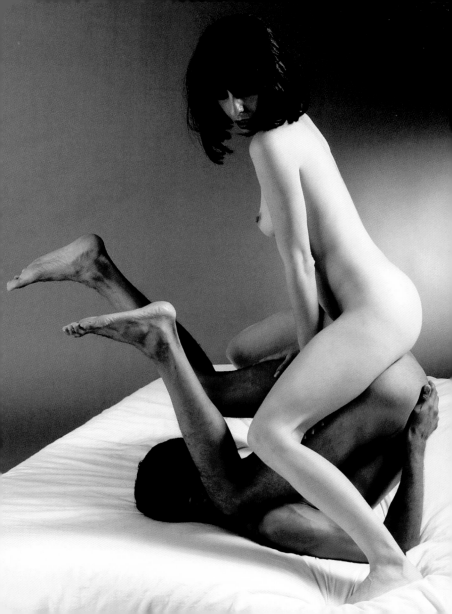

267

Riding into the Sunset

The man lies on his back on the bed and pushes his bottom up off the bed (like an old-fashioned bicycle exercise) and lifts his legs, bringing his knees toward his chest. She straddles his body and slides down onto his erect penis. She then bends and straightens her knees, controlling the thrusts.

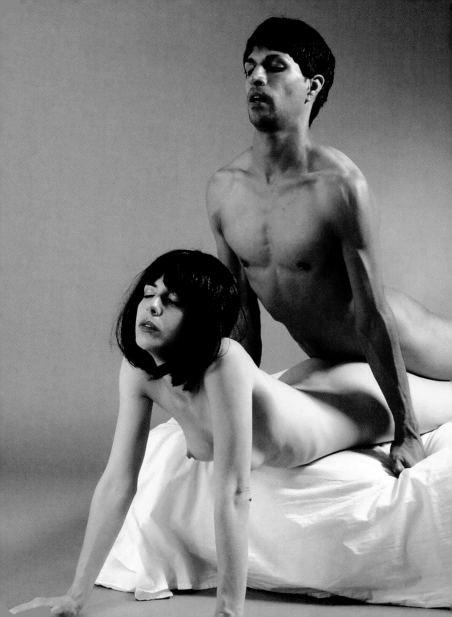

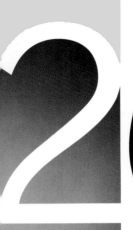
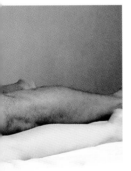
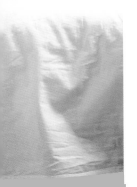

268

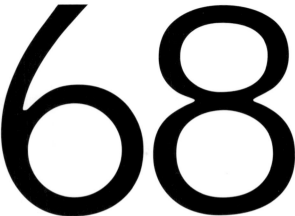

The Alligator

She lies on bed with her top half hanging off facing the floor, using her hands on the floor to support her. He enters her anally and holds his upper half off of her so that their top halves are at a 90-degree angle.

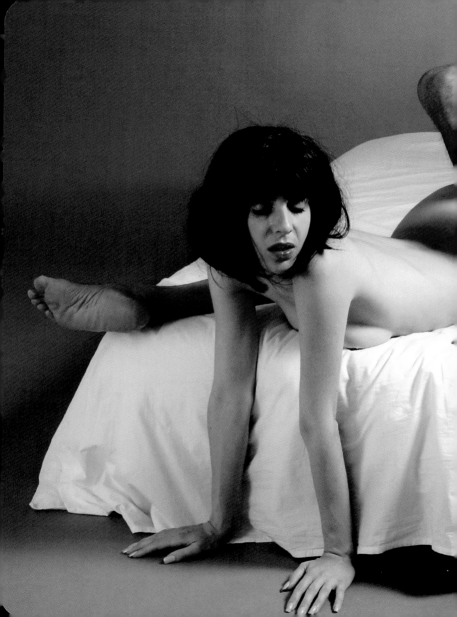

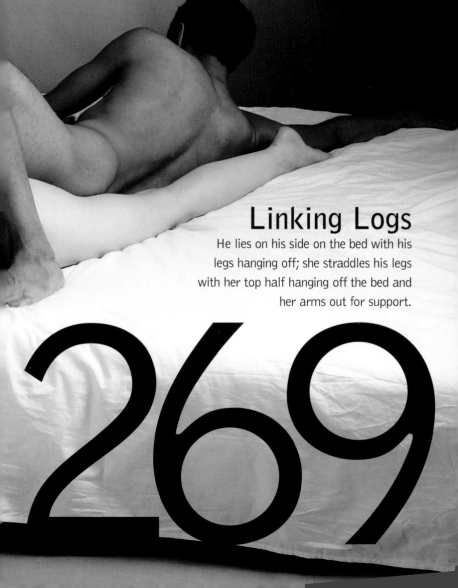

Linking Logs

He lies on his side on the bed with his legs hanging off; she straddles his legs with her top half hanging off the bed and her arms out for support.

269

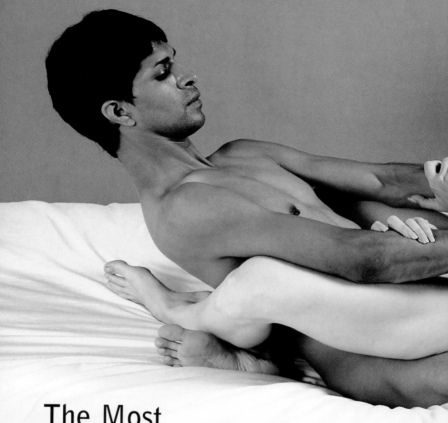

The Most
Beautiful Flower

He sits on the bed slightly away from edge, and she sits
on him and slides herself onto his penis. She wraps legs
around his bottom, and he holds her by the forearms as
she relaxes and reclines almost to the floor, and he pulls
her toward him and slowly lets her fall away.

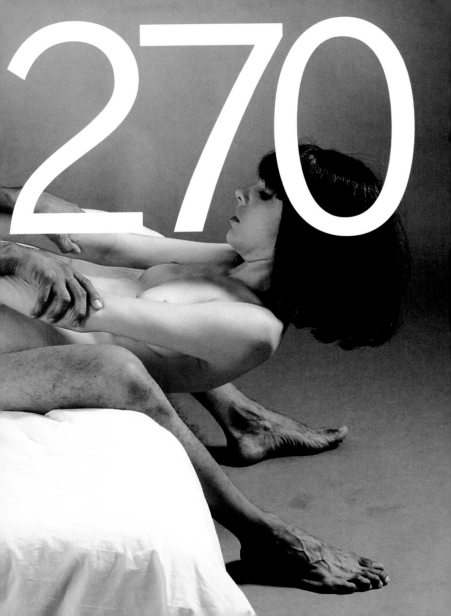

270

271

The Contortionist

She starts on all fours and proceeds to rest on her shoulder and head. The man squats above her, penetrating her well-lubed anus and using her as a seat in this unusual and unusually pleasing position.

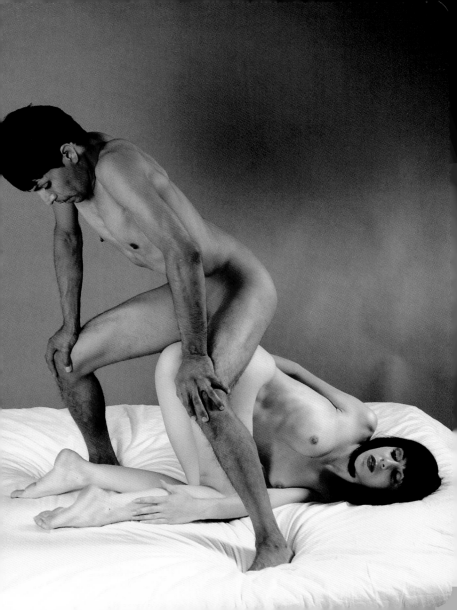

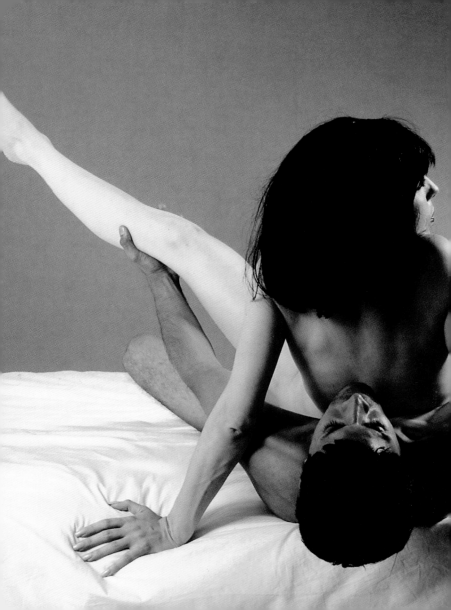

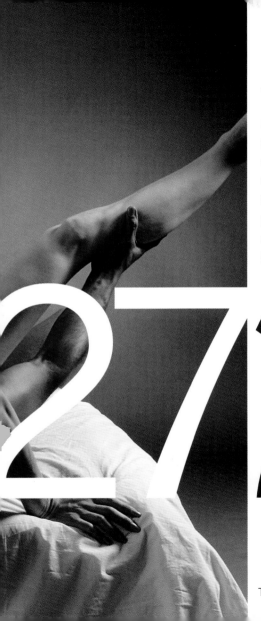

The Cricket

He lies on his back on the bed with knees bent and to the side; she lies on top of him with her back to him, and he holds her legs spread open and penetrates from behind. He is able to squeeze her legs closed for a tighter fit.

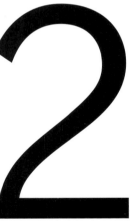

272

273

Flambé

He lies on his back on the bed and holds his left leg up and out in contact with her right hip; she kneels in between his legs and rides him while both garnish each other with chocolate body paint.

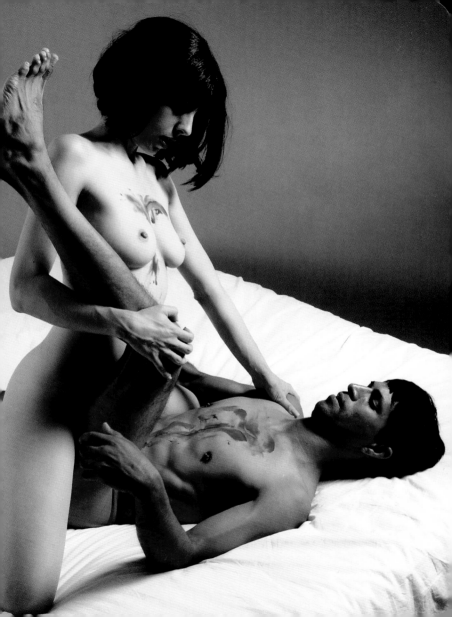

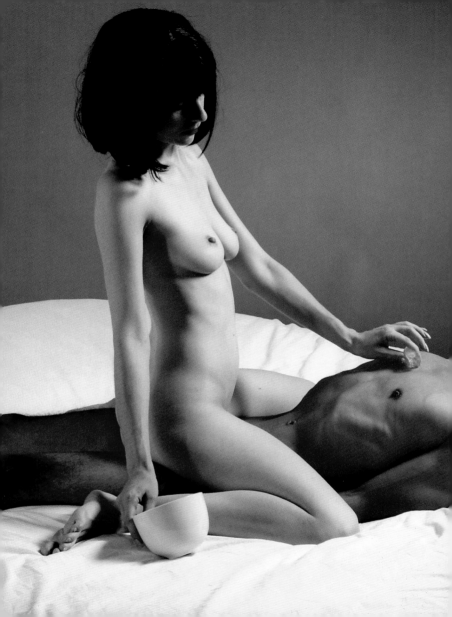

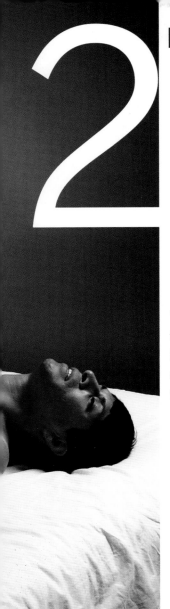

274

Hottest Snow

The man lies on his back on the bed; the woman straddles and sits on his penis, her legs bent under her. They massage each other with ice cubes to quench their fiery passion for just a moment.

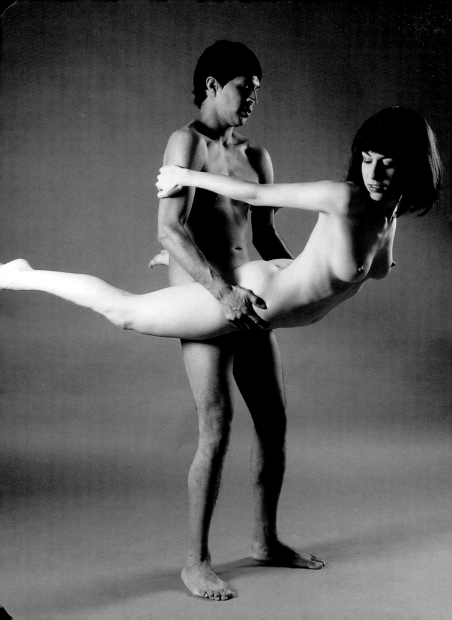

275

Vroom, Vroom

As his lover lies facedown on the bed, the man should penetrate her while standing behind her, and lift her by the hips as she grasps onto his arms for support as she orgasms in the air.

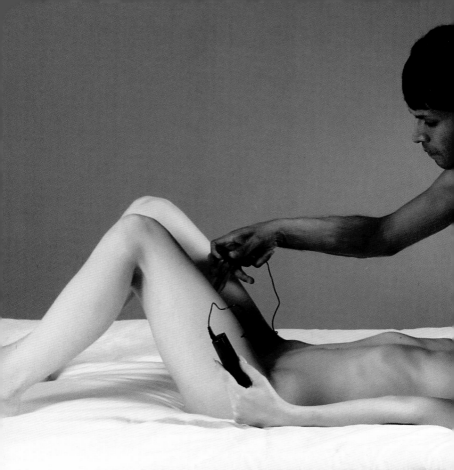

Section Twelve:
Advanced Toys

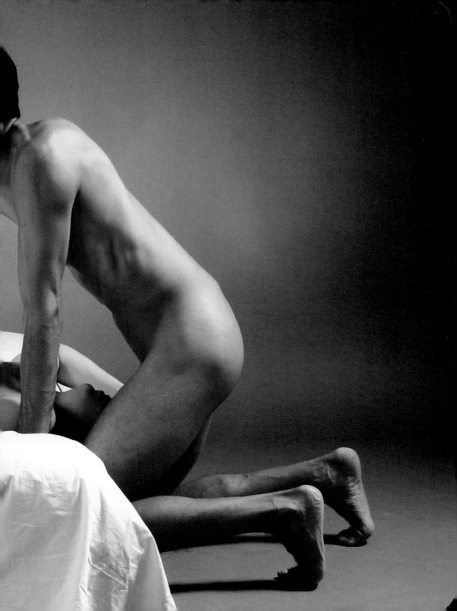

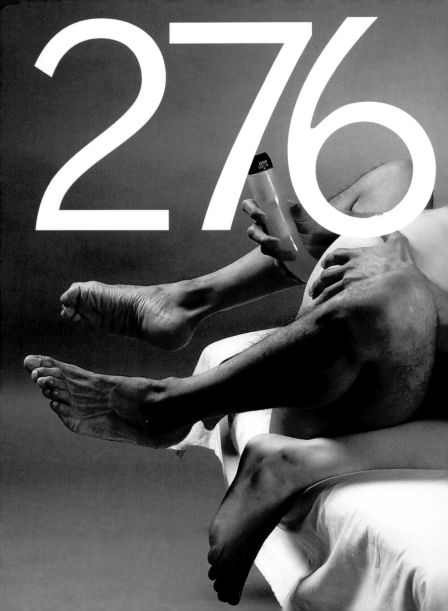

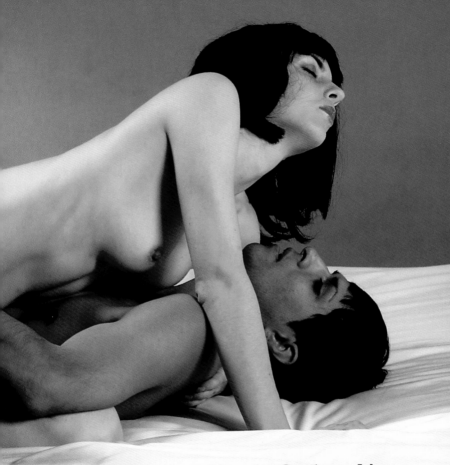

From Both Sides Now

Lying on the edge of the bed, the man takes the
woman on top of him and uses a toy to anally
penetrate her as he enters her vaginally.

277

Good Vibrations

She sits on edge of bed with a dildo; he bends forward, resting his hands on his knees. She penetrates with the dildo and perhaps stimulates his penis manually.

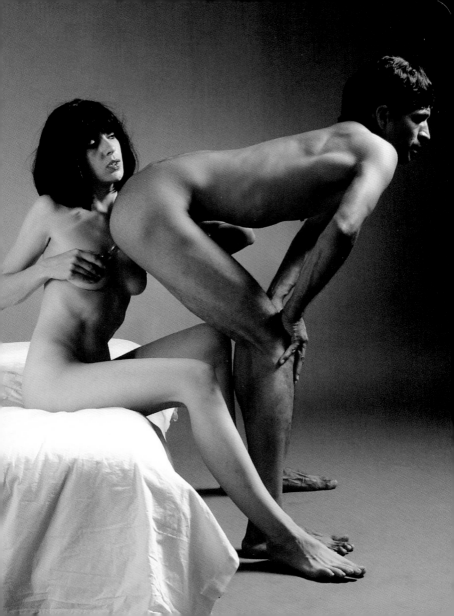

278

Hugging the Pole

The woman lies on her right side on the bed and pulls one leg up into the air (like a half-split); man kneels in front of her and rubs his penis against her raised leg, and she rests her leg on his shoulder; he inserts a dildo into her and strokes both.

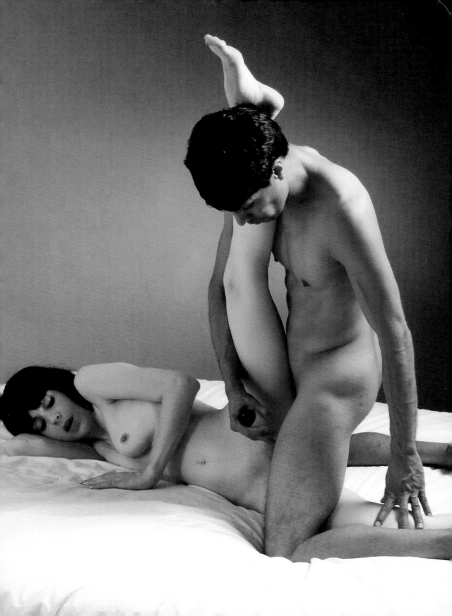

279

Missile Launcher

A quick move from Fighter Planes (266), the woman uses her left hand to insert an anal plug, allowing him to feel weightless and grounded at the same moment.

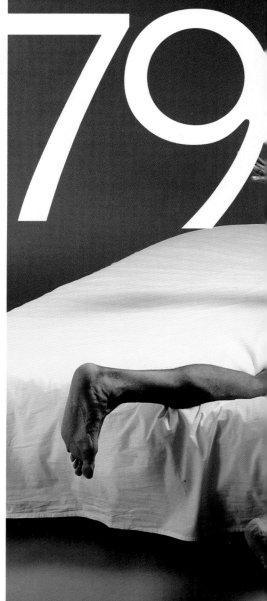

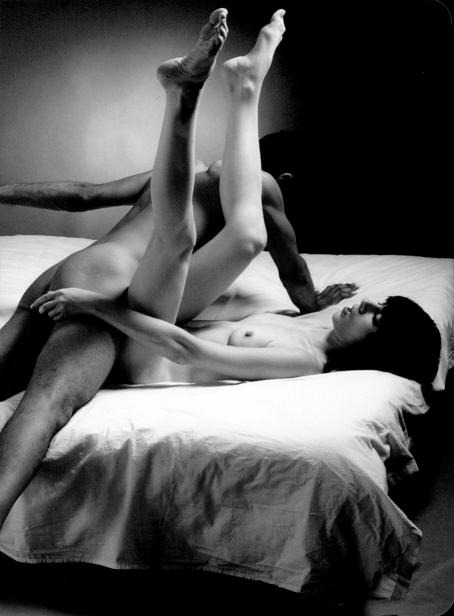

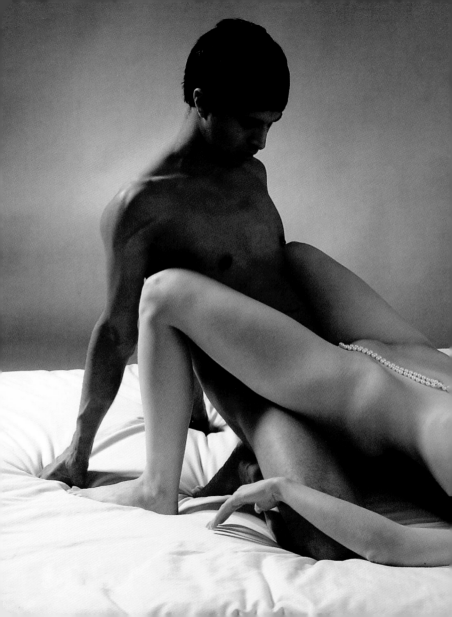

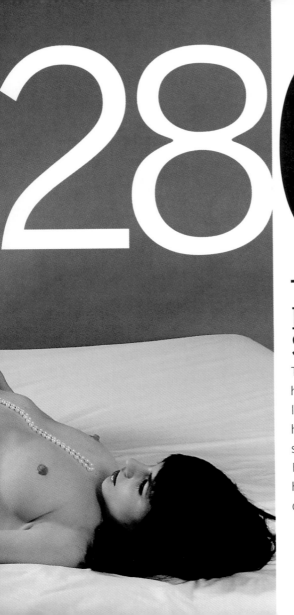

280

The Impaled Seesaw

The man leans back on his knees and enters his lover anally, as she inserts her string of pearls and stimulates her clitoris. He supports himself on his fists and pulls the toy out slowly as they climax.

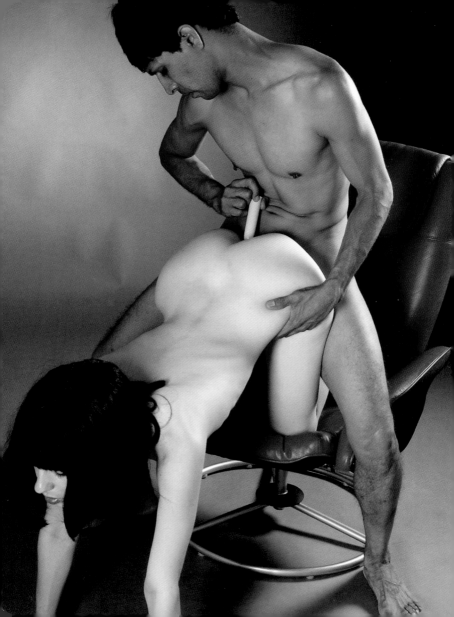

281

Pulling the Plug

A quick movement from Under Wraps (230), here the man flips the woman onto her stomach, and uses a toy to doubly penetrate her, adding to the sensual experience for both of them.

282

Watch Out Behind You

Resting one lifted leg on the chair, the woman opens herself up for deep penetration with a toy. The man is free to move all around her, creating immense pleasure without having to remain stationary.

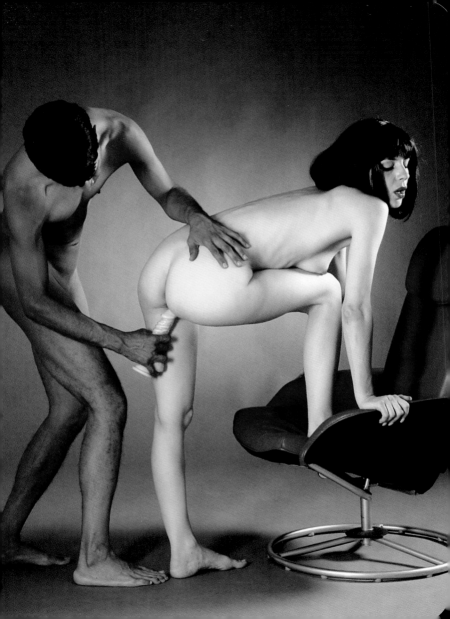

283

Acrobatics

The woman sits on a chair with the man lying below her. He brings her to orgasm using toys and his fingers, and she is free to watch from above. Her hands are loose to support her, or assist him by stimulating herself.

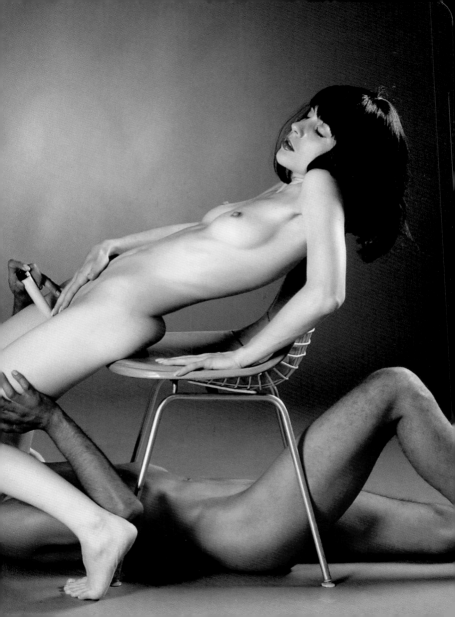

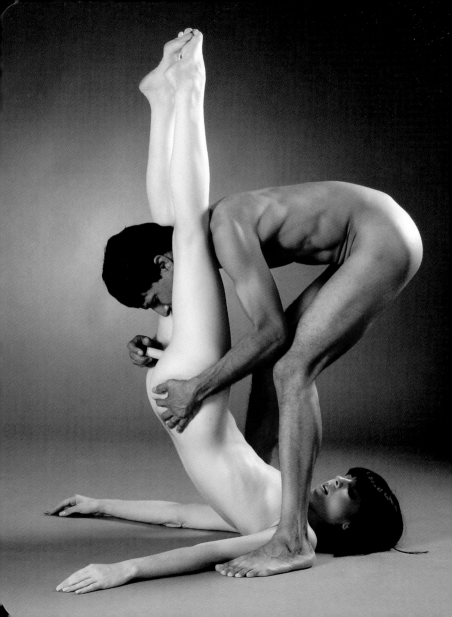

284

The Gladiator's Torch

Moving from The Circle of Pleasure (208),
the man enters the woman with a toy, leaving his
mouth free to kiss up and down her legs, as he
continues supporting her torso.

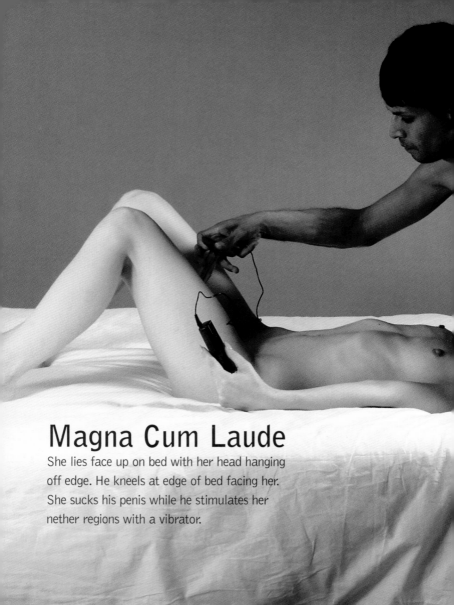

Magna Cum Laude

She lies face up on bed with her head hanging
off edge. He kneels at edge of bed facing her.
She sucks his penis while he stimulates her
nether regions with a vibrator.

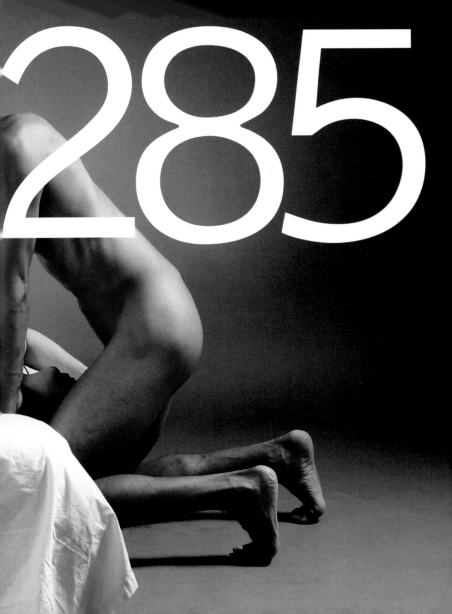

285

Section Thirteen:
Swing Time!

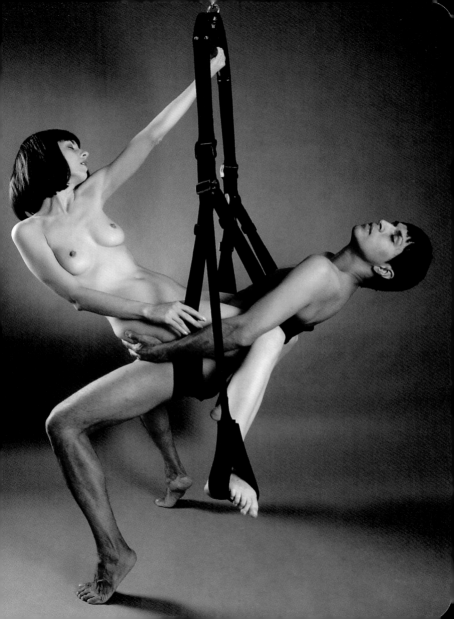

286

The Shrieking Monkey

Practically weightless, the woman goes bananas as she swings freely back and forth onto her lover's tongue. He can alternate between manual and oral stimulation until she is shrieking with orgasm.

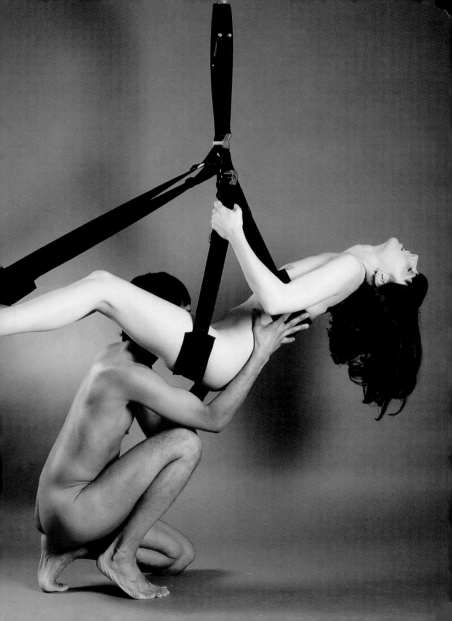

287

Sweet Chariot

The man stands while the woman crouches in the swing in front of him. This allows for deep penetration and a combination of bouncing and thrusting, all of which the man can enjoy without the overexertion related to lifting his partner.

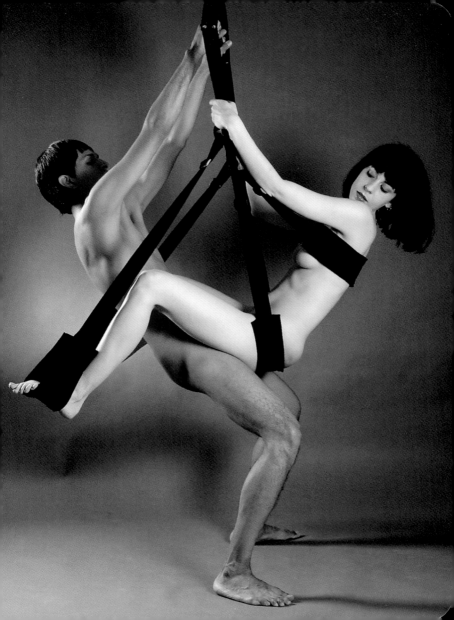

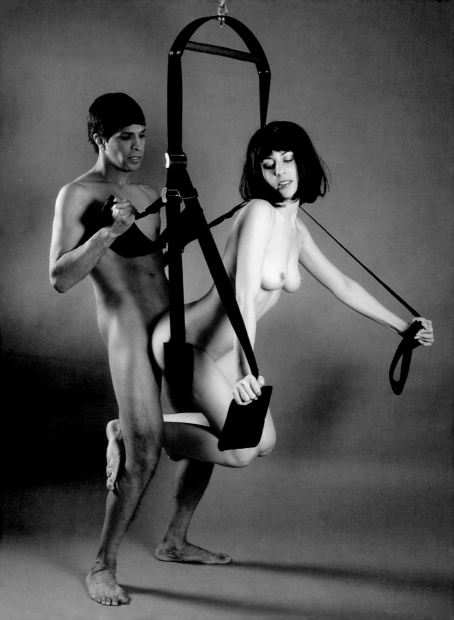

288

Get Sprung

The woman sticks out her gorgeous behind, and is anally or vaginally penetrated from behind while the man stands, able to grip any part of her or the swing itself. As in Sweet Chariot (287), each can fully enjoy bouncing and thrusting without worry of strain.

289

The Rocking Cradle

As the man sits in the swing, the woman lowers herself onto him, feeling every long inch of him in all new places as each leans back and rock gently, suspended and weightless.

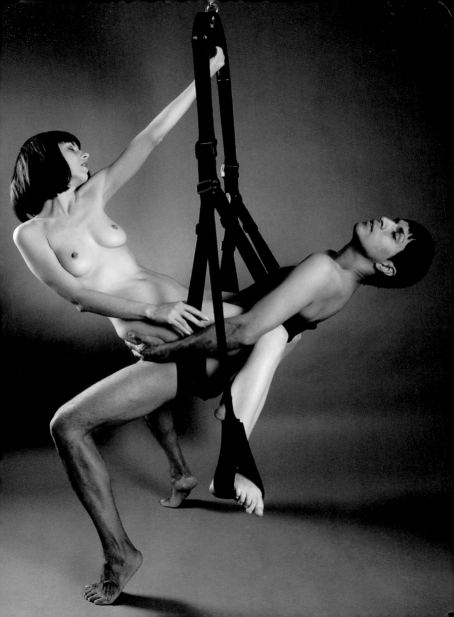

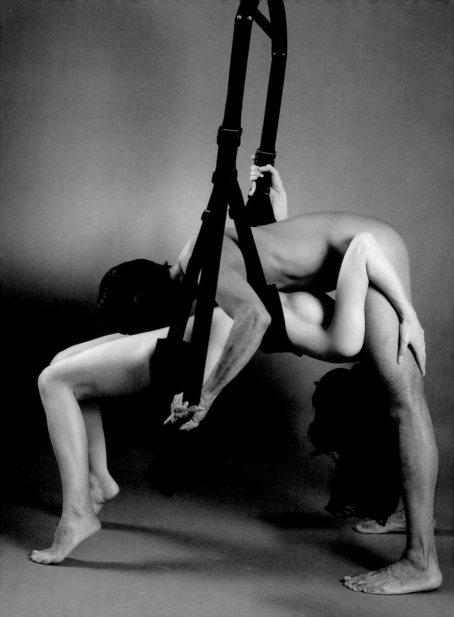

290

Dinner for Two

With no worries of smothering the bottom partner, the couple engages in mutually beneficial oral sex. They bring each other to climax while swaying gently, enjoying the feel of air all over their bodies.

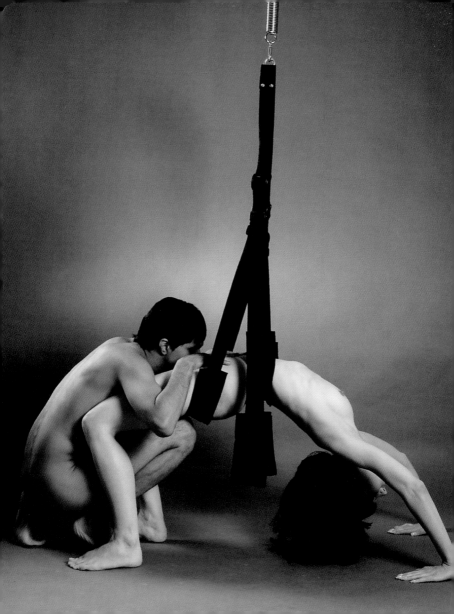

291

Dinner for One

The woman arches her back in comfortable ecstasy, using her arms to control her pleasure level. The man crouches with his partner's feet planted on the floor or her legs draped over his shoulders, enjoying his meal.

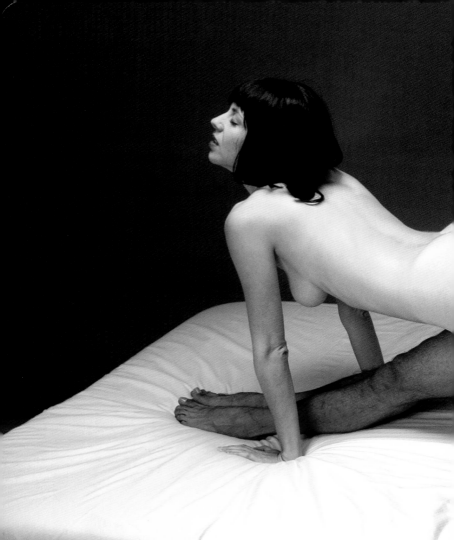

Checklist

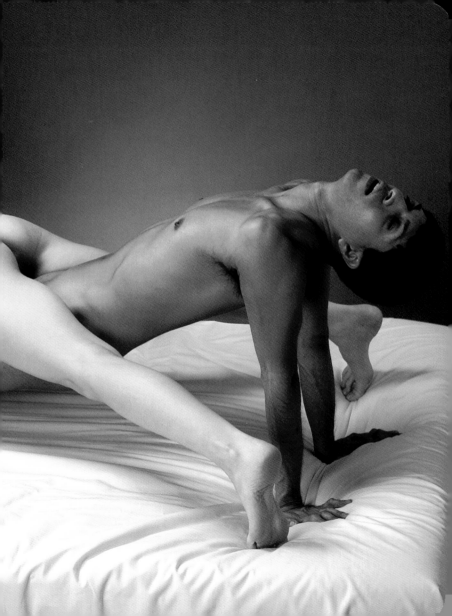

Checklist

This handy checklist is useful in many ways. Not only does it give you a thumbnail visual of each position for quick reference, but it also allows you to keep track of the positions as you enjoy them. Or, be creative and make icons for your favorite positons, easy positions, and positions that will take some yoga classes to master!

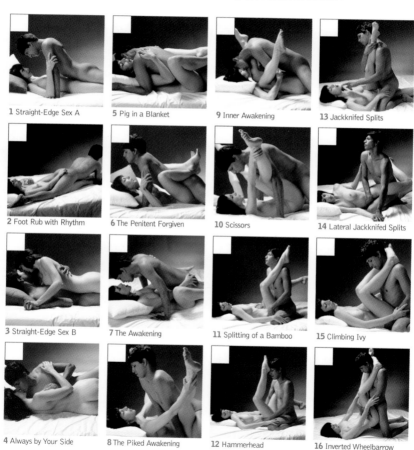

1 Straight-Edge Sex A

5 Pig in a Blanket

9 Inner Awakening

13 Jackknifed Splits

2 Foot Rub with Rhythm

6 The Penitent Forgiven

10 Scissors

14 Lateral Jackknifed Splits

3 Straight-Edge Sex B

7 The Awakening

11 Splitting of a Bamboo

15 Climbing Ivy

4 Always by Your Side

8 The Piked Awakening

12 Hammerhead

16 Inverted Wheelbarrow

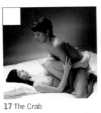
17 The Crab

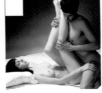
22 Side-to-Side Press

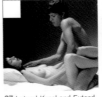
27 Lateral Kneel and Extend

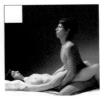
32 Pelvic Lap Dance

18 The Wrapped Crab

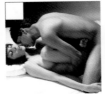
23 Half Lotus

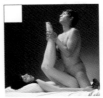
28 Kneel and Push Back

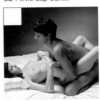
33 Locked Lap Dance

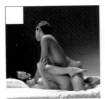
19 The Open Crab

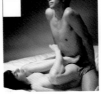
24 Full Lotus

29 Side-to-Side Kneel and Extend

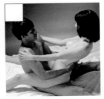
34 Kama's Wheel

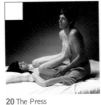
20 The Press

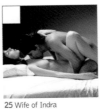
25 Wife of Indra

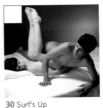
30 Surf's Up

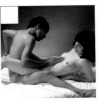
35 Reclining Kama's Wheel

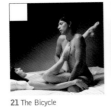
21 The Bicycle

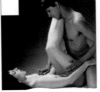
26 Kneel and Extend

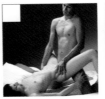
31 Pelvic Thrust

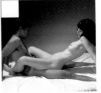
36 Snake Trap

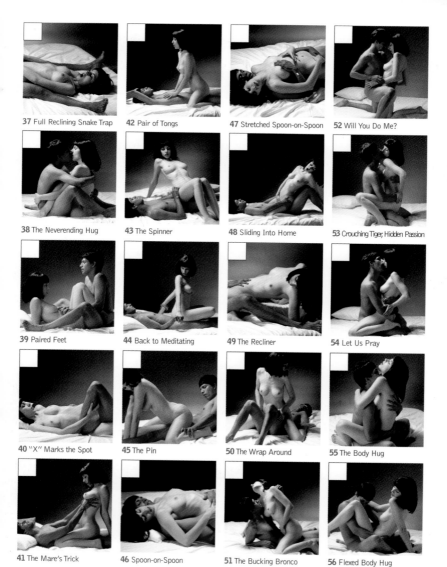

37 Full Reclining Snake Trap

42 Pair of Tongs

47 Stretched Spoon-on-Spoon

52 Will You Do Me?

38 The Neverending Hug

43 The Spinner

48 Sliding Into Home

53 Crouching Tiger, Hidden Passion

39 Paired Feet

44 Back to Meditating

49 The Recliner

54 Let Us Pray

40 "X" Marks the Spot

45 The Pin

50 The Wrap Around

55 The Body Hug

41 The Mare's Trick

46 Spoon-on-Spoon

51 The Bucking Bronco

56 Flexed Body Hug

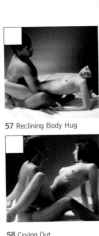

57 Reclining Body Hug

58 Crying Out

59 Sweet Abandon

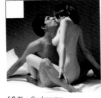

60 The Corkscrew

61 The Flexed Corkscrew

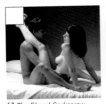

62 Inverted Headlock

63 The See-Saw A

64 The See-Saw B

65 The Backbend A

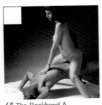

66 The Throne

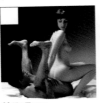

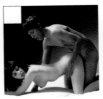

67 See Spot Come

68 The Dutch Doggy

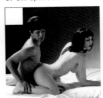

69 Taking Sides

70 The Back Scratcher

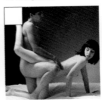

71 Enveloped in Love

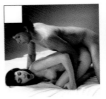

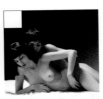

72 Baby Elephant

73 Open Elephant

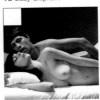

74 The Elephant

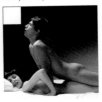

75 Sitting Body Wrap

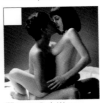

76 Sitting Flexed Body Wrap

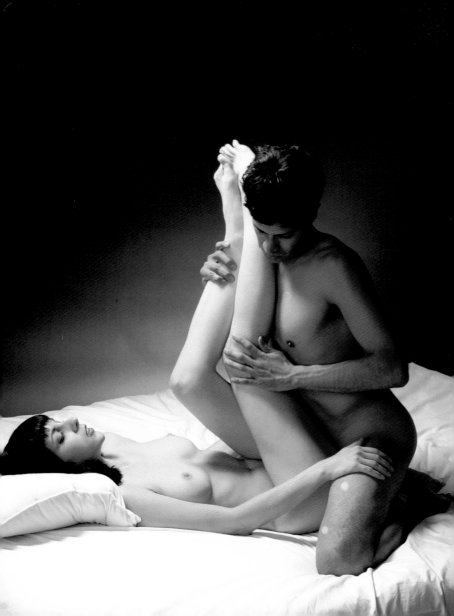

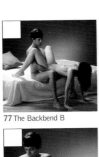
77 The Backbend B

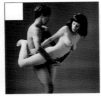
82 Stand by Your Man

87 The Hoover

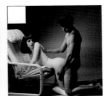
92 Purrfect Plunge

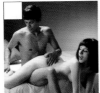
78 The Pushover

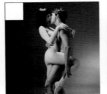
83 The Tango

88 The Hoover Upright

93 The Lounge Cat

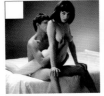
79 The Cobra

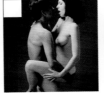
84 The Harness

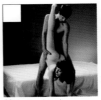
89 The Handstand

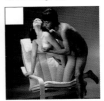
94 Fido's on His Feet

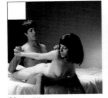
80 The Pilot

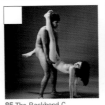
85 The Backbend C

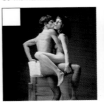
90 The Leg Up

95 The Wheelbarrow

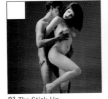
81 The Stick Up

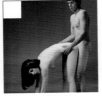
86 Congress of the Cow

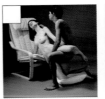
91 The Chair Lift

96 Lay-Z Girl

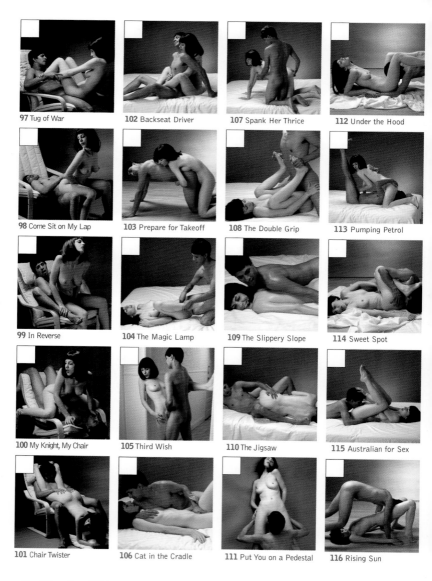

97 Tug of War

102 Backseat Driver

107 Spank Her Thrice

112 Under the Hood

98 Come Sit on My Lap

103 Prepare for Takeoff

108 The Double Grip

113 Pumping Petrol

99 In Reverse

104 The Magic Lamp

109 The Slippery Slope

114 Sweet Spot

100 My Knight, My Chair

105 Third Wish

110 The Jigsaw

115 Australian for Sex

101 Chair Twister

106 Cat in the Cradle

111 Put You on a Pedestal

116 Rising Sun

117 The Dip

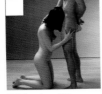
122 Downtown Girl

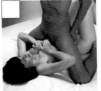
127 Tunnel of Love

132 My Door Is Always Open

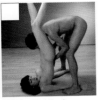
118 The Bird Feeder

123 Slippery When Wet

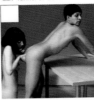
128 Checking the Oil

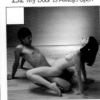
133 The Nexus

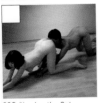
119 Chasing the Cat

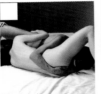
124 Always on Your Side

129 Bumper Cars

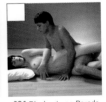
134 Elephants on Parade

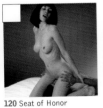
120 Seat of Honor

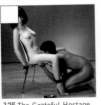
125 The Grateful Hostage

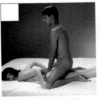
130 Back in the Saddle

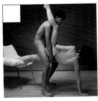
135 Table Saw

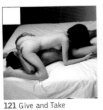
121 Give and Take

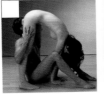
126 A Bridge to Pleasure

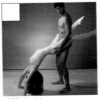
131 The Plow

136 Queen of the World

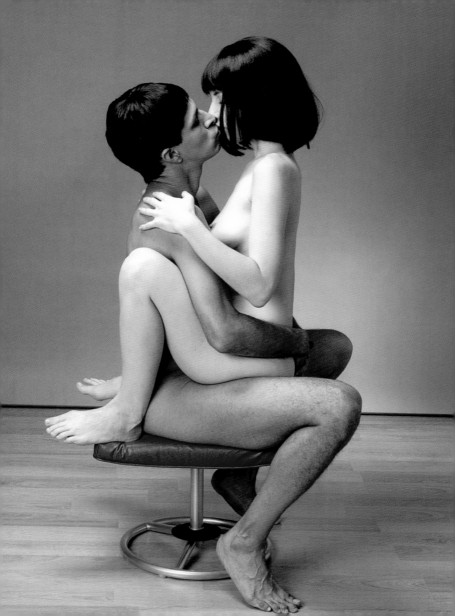

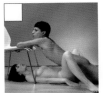 137 Fantasy City

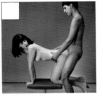 142 Lean on Me

 147 Tight Quarters

 152 Climbing the Walls

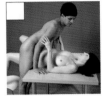 138 The Dinner Party

 143 The Consolation

 148 I've Found My Niche

 153 Synchronized Deep Diving

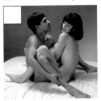 139 The Kissing Lotus

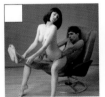 144 Lady Godiva

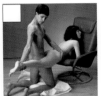 149 The Long and Deep of It

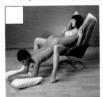 154 Long Night, Full Moon

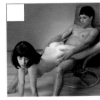 140 The Sheath

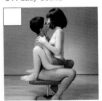 145 Bare Hug

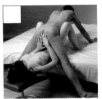 150 Into Each, His Own

 155 Spreading Some Joy

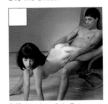 141 Members Only Entrance

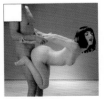 146 Cupid's Bow

 151 The Door Jam

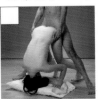 156 Deep Satisfaction

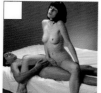 **157** Surfing the Wave

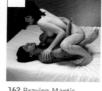 **162** Praying Mantis

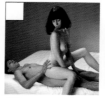 **167** Hopping the Fence

 172 Working Your Way Up

 158 Leapfrog

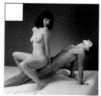 **163** Lowered Inhibition

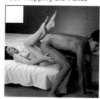 **168** I Saved Your Seat

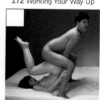 **173** Out of the Box

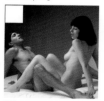 **159** Blooming Lotus

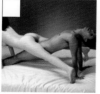 **164** Meet Me in the Middle

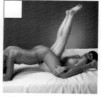 **169** Upside Down You Turn Me

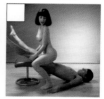 **174** Power Broker

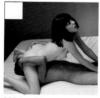 **160** Speaking in Tongues

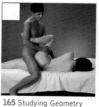 **165** Studying Geometry

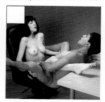 **170** The Corporate Merger

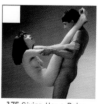 **175** Giving Her a Raise

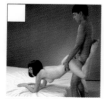 **161** The Nail-Gun

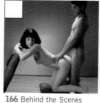 **166** Behind the Scenes

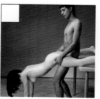 **171** The Motivator

 176 Entry-Level Position

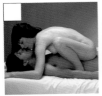 **177** Loving Takeover

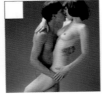 **182** The Profit Share

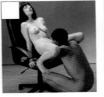 **187** Appealing to Your…

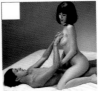 **192** Performance Art

 178 Climbing the Ladder

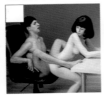 **183** Take a Letter Please

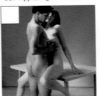 **188** Better Than Phone Sex

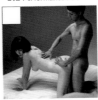 **193** Smear Tactics

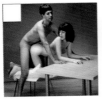 **179** Behind on Work

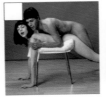 **184** Sharing Your Assets

 189 Tight Schedule

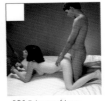 **194** Prisoner of Love

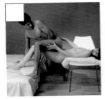 **180** Flex Benefits

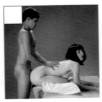 **185** Squeeze Me In

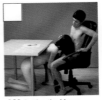 **190** Getting the Memo

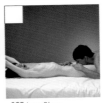 **195** Love Slave

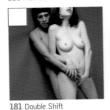 **181** Double Shift

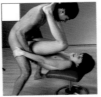 **186** Ruthless Negotiator

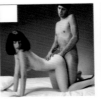 **191** Rough Rider

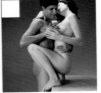 **196** Impaled Passion

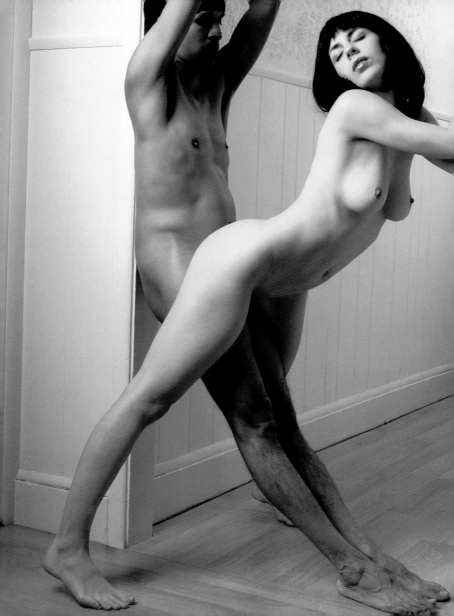

197 Working Every Angle

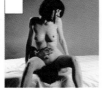 202 Eating In

 207 The Ben Dover

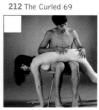 212 The Curled 69

 198 Trapped Bumblebee

 203 Stand and Deliver

 208 The Circle of Pleasure

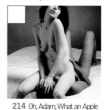 213 Slap and Tickle

 198 Fire and Ice

 204 Nose to the Grindstone

 209 Kiss My . . .

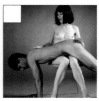 214 Oh, Adam, What an Apple

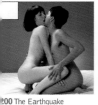 200 The Earthquake

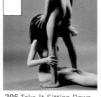 205 Take It Sitting Down

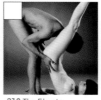 210 The Elevator

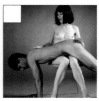 215 Give Him a Hand

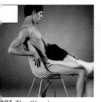 201 The Classic

 206 The Happy Puppy

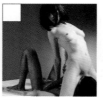 211 The Landscape of Two Mountains

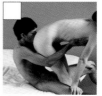 216 O Marks the Spot

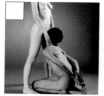
217 Mistress May I?

222 Learning to Walk

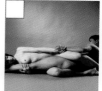
227 The Intertwined Links

232 Rock-a-Bye Baby

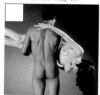
218 The Sack of Potatoes

223 The Golden Eagle

228 Chain Me Up

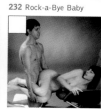
233 The Curling Iron

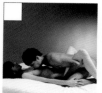
219 The Cradle

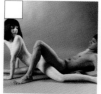
224 Crossing the River

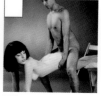
229 Shucking the Oyster

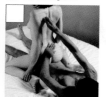
234 Like a Cat

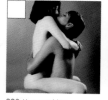
220 Hammocking

225 The Carriage House

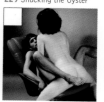
230 Under Wraps

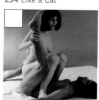
235 On the Road

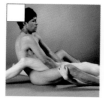
221 Salted or Unsalted?

226 Catch You on the Flip Side

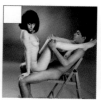
231 The Kitchen Sink

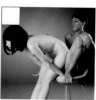
236 The Whoopie Cushion

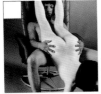
237 Sailor's Knots

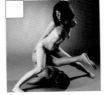
242 Doing Cartwheels

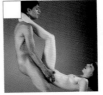
247 Roll Your Rs

252 Ice Hot

238 The Cancan Dancer

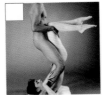
243 The Headstand...

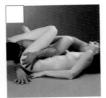
248 That's a Wrap

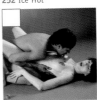
253 What's for Dessert?

239 The Venus Flytrap

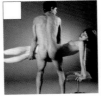
244 Pole Vaulting

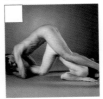
249 Mountain's Majesty

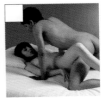
254 Sole-ful

240 The Homestretch

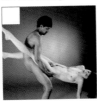
245 Springing

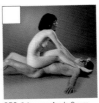
250 Crisscross Apple Sauce

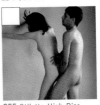
255 Stiletto High-Rise

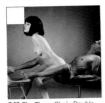
241 The Three-Chair Double Squat

246 The Plow and Hoe

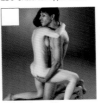
251 Welcome Home

256 See You Later

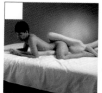
257 The Great Plains

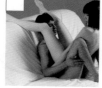
262 Rolling Hills

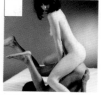
267 Riding into the Sunset

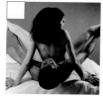
272 The Cricket

258 For Your Thighs Only

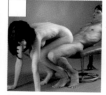
263 Ready, Set, Go!

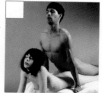
268 The Alligator

273 Flambé

259 Sandy Dunes

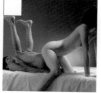
264 The Black Spider

269 Linking Logs

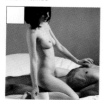
274 Hottest Snow

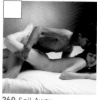
260 Sail Away

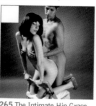
265 The Intimate Hip Grasp

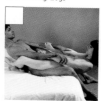
270 The Most Beautiful Flower

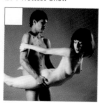
275 Vroom, Vroom

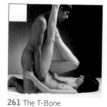
261 The T-Bone

266 Fighter Planes

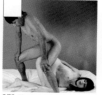
271 The Contortionist

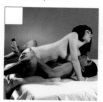
276 From Both Sides Now

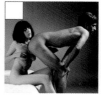 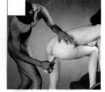 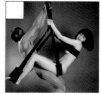

277 Good Vibrations   **282** Watch Out Behind You   **287** Sweet Chariot

 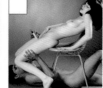 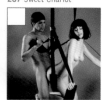

278 Hugging the Pole   **283** Acrobatics   **288** Get Sprung

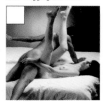 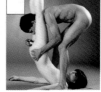 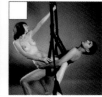

279 Missle Launcher   **284** The Gladiator's Torch   **289** The Rocking Cradle

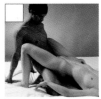 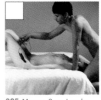 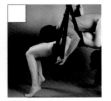

280 The Impaled Seesaw   **285** Magna Cum Laude   **290** Dinner for Two

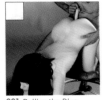 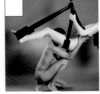 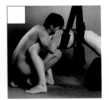

281 Pulling the Plug   **286** The Shrieking Monkey   **291** Dinner for One